MENTAL ILLNESS AND SOCIAL POLICY

THE AMERICAN EXPERIENCE

MENTAL ILLNESS AND SOCIAL POLICY

THE AMERICAN EXPERIENCE

Advisory Editor
GERALD N. GROB

Editorial Board
ERIC T. CARLSON
BLANCHE D. COLL
CHARLES E. ROSENBERG

THE BEGINNINGS

of

AMERICAN PSYCHIATRIC THOUGHT

and

PRACTICE

Five Accounts, 1811-1830

ARNO PRESS
A NEW YORK TIMES COMPANY
New York • 1973

Reprint Edition 1973 by Arno Press Inc.

MENTAL ILLNESS AND SOCIAL POLICY:
   The American Experience
ISBN for complete set: 0-405-05190-5
See last pages of this volume for titles.

Manufactured in the United States of America

Library of Congress Cataloging in Publication Data
Main entry under title.

The Beginnings of American psychiatric thought and
   practice.

   (Mental illness and social policy: the American
experience)
   Reprint of Account of the rise and progress of the
asylum, first published by Kimber and Conrad,
Philadelphia, 1814; of An inaugural dissertation on
insanity, by T. R. Beck, first published New York, 1811;
of Hints for introducing an improved mode of treating
the insane in the asylum, by T. Eddy, first published
New York, 1815; of Proposals for establishing a retreat
for the insane, by G. Parkman, first published Boston,
1814; of A discourse on mental philosophy as connected
with mental disease, by R. Wyman, first published Boston,
1830.
   1. Psychiatry--Early works to 1900--Addresses,
essays, lectures.   I. Series.   [DNLM: WM B416
1830F]
RC340.B4 1973   616.8'9'00973   73-2384
ISBN 0-405-05192-1

Contents

ACCOUNT

OF

THE RISE AND PROGRESS

OF

THE ASYLUM

ACCOUNT

OF

THE RISE AND PROGRESS

OF

THE ASYLUM,

Proposed to be Established, near Philadelphia,

FOR THE

RELIEF OF PERSONS

DEPRIVED OF THE USE OF THEIR REASON,

WITH AN

ABRIDGED ACCOUNT

OF

THE RETREAT,

A SIMILAR INSTITUTION NEAR YORK, IN ENGLAND

PHILADELPHIA:
PUBLISHED BY KIMBER AND CONRAD,
No. 93. MARKET STREET.
Conrad, Printer.

1814.

ACCOUNT, &c.

AT the annual meeting of the Contributors to the Asylum for the Relief of Persons deprived of the use of their Reason, held in the Third Month, 1814, an Account of the Rise and Progress of the Institution was directed to be published, for the information of Friends.

PROPOSALS were made to the Yearly Meeting in 1811, from two of the Quarterly Meetings, "to make provision for such of our members as may be deprived of the use of their reason;" the consideration of which subject being referred to a committee, they made a report thereon; which was adopted by the meeting in the succeeding year. And the following plan and proposals were spread amongst Friends in consequence of this conclusion.

PLAN OF AN ASYLUM,

For the Relief of Persons deprived of the use of their Reason.

THE Committee appointed by the Yearly Meeting, held at Philadelphia, to take under consideration the subject respecting a provision

for such of our members as may be deprived
of the use of their Reason, reported,

" That, considering the peculiar circumstances of this afflicted class of our members, as
well as the relief of their families and friends,
they believed that the establishment proposed,
under direction of such members of our Yearly
Meeting as might be willing to contribute there-
to, would be beneficial."

And the Yearly Meeting having adopted this
Report, in the Fourth Month last, a number
of Friends met at Philadelphia to deliberate on
the most suitable means of carrying the same
into effect. They have accordingly agreed upon
a Plan, and form of Subscription Papers, the
distribution of which was committed to the following Friends :

Thomas Scattergood,	*Emmor Kimber,*
Jonathan Evans,	*Thomas Wistar,*
Ellis Yarnall,	*Samuel Powel Griffitts.*
Isaac Bonsall,	

It appears very desirable that an institution
should be formed, in a retired situation, with
the necessary medical assistance, and wholly
under the care and notice of Friends, for the
relief and accommodation of persons thus afflicted ; including members and professors with
us, of every description, with respect to property. This would serve to alleviate the anxiety of their relatives, to tranquillize the minds
of the afflicted in their lucid intervals, and
would, moreover, tend to facilitate their recovery.

It is therefore proposed, that, if proper encouragement be given, a sufficient quantity of

land be purchased near Philadelphia, and a building erected thereon, which may accommodate, at least, fifty persons.

The institution to be established and supported by legacies, donations, and subscriptions; to be promoted amongst Friends.

Any Monthly Meeting, belonging to our Yearly Meeting, contributing two hundred dollars, and every individual subscribing ten dollars per annum, or fifty dollars at one time; being and continuing a member of our religious society, shall be considered members of the institution.

All annual subscriptions under ten dollars, or sums contributed under fifty dollars, shall be considered as donations.

The members shall meet, annually, at Philadelphia, on the fourth day preceding the third Sixth-day of the week, in the Third Month, and choose, from amongst the subscribers, members of our Yearly Meeting, twenty persons as a committee to manage all the affairs of the institution. At these annual meetings, a report of the last year's proceedings shall be produced by the committee. Every Monthly Meeting contributing as above, shall have the right of appointing an agent, who may appear and act on their behalf at these meetings.

Every Monthly Meeting which has contributed two hundred dollars, and every individual who has contributed fifty dollars, whilst continuing a member of our religious society, may recommend one poor patient, at one time, on the lowest terms of admission.

It is believed that the establishment of an institution of this kind will meet with the gene-

A 2

ral approbation of Friends; and they are accordingly invited to contribute their aid, as it embraces all classes of the society, and is meant to afford relief in one of the most distressing maladies that human nature is subject to.

The first general meeting of the subscribers will be held in Philadelphia, at the Mulberry Street meeting house, at seven o'clock in the evening, on the fourth day of the week preceding the next Yearly Meeting.

JONATHAN EVANS, of Philadelphia, will receive the contributions until a treasurer is appointed.

Philadelphia, Twelfth Month, 5th, 1812.

In pursuance of these proposals, the first Meeting of the Contributors was held in Philadelphia, on the fourteenth day of the Fourth Month 1813, and at the next meeting in the Sixth Month, the following Constitution was adopted.

CONSTITUTION.

We the subscribers, members of the Yearly Meeting of Friends held in Philadelphia, desirous to provide for the suitable accommodation of that afflicted class of our fellow members and professors with us, who are or may be deprived of the use of their reason, as well as the relief of their families and friends; have associated for the purpose of establishing an Asylum for their reception, which is intended to furnish, besides the requisite medical aid, such tender sympathetic attention and religious oversight, as may soothe their agitated minds and thereby, under the divine blessing, facilitate their restoration to the enjoyment of this inestimable gift. For which purpose the following articles of association have been agreed upon.

ARTICLE I.

The Association shall be known by the name and title of "the Contributors to the Asylum for the Relief of persons deprived of the use of their Reason."

ARTICLE II.

Any Monthly Meeting belonging to the Yearly Meeting of Friends held in Philadelphia, contributing two hundred dollars, and every individual subscribing ten dollars per annum, or fifty dollars at one time, and being and continuing members of the Religious Society of Friends, shall be considered members of this Association; and a Monthly Meeting so contributing, shall have the right to appoint an agent, who may appear and act at the meetings of the Association on their behalf.

ARTICLE III.

The contributors shall meet annually, at Philadelphia, on the Fourth-day preceding the third Sixth-day of the week in the Third Month, and choose from amongst themselves twenty Managers, a Treasurer and Clerk; who shall continue in office for one year, and until others shall be appointed. They shall also transact at this meeting such business of the Institution as may appear necessary.

ARTICLE IV.

The Managers shall meet at least once in every month, and eleven of them shall be a board to transact business. They shall appoint one of their number to act as Clerk. They shall choose and appoint the physicians : they shall also appoint the superintendant and matron of the Asylum, and prescribe their duties, and shall have the controul of all other officers and assistants whom it may be necessary to emp'oy in the service of the Institution. They shall fix the salaries of the persons employed, and the rates to be paid for patients; and all monies drawn from the Treasurer shall be by their order, and signed by the Clerk, which orders shall be his vouchers. They shall make such rules and regulations for the domestic and general government of the establishment, as may from time to time appear requisite. The minutes of their proceedings, with a summary statement thereof, shall be laid before the contributors at their annual meeting in the Third Month. They may call special meetings of the association, whenever, in their judgment, it appears necessary.

ARTICLE V.

The Treasurer shall receive all the monies of the Institution, and pay them to the orders of the Board of Managers ; who shall examine and settle his accounts, and produce the same to the annual meeting of the Association in the Third Month. He shall keep regular accounts, to be

at all times subject to the inspection of the
Board of Managers.

ARTICLE VI.

Every Monthly Meeting which has contributed two hundred dollars, and every individual
who has contributed fifty dollars in one payment,
whilst continuing a member of the religious society of Friends, may recommend one poor patient at one time on the lowest terms of admission. Application for admission shall be made
first to one of the Physicians for examination,
and then to the Managers; or to such of them
as they may appoint for that purpose, by whom
all orders for admission shall be granted; and
when they find it difficult to agree on the propriety of admitting the applicant, the case shall
be referred to the decision of the Board of
Managers.

ARTICLE VII.

The estate of the Contributors, acquired for
the purposes of this Institution, shall be conveyed to twelve of their number to be held in trust,
who shall be appointed at an annual or special
meeting of the Association.

ARTICLE VIII.

No alteration in these Articles shall be made
except at a stated Annual Meeting of the Association. And no change shall at any time be
made which shall infringe on the right hereby
vested in Monthly Meetings, or individuals, to

recommend patients on the lowest terms of admission.

A tract of land about five miles distant from Philadelphia, and one mile westward of Frankford, containing fifty two acres, has been purchased, and the premises conveyed to twelve of the Contributors in trust for the Institution. The land is of good quality, in an high and healthy situation, with a considerable proportion of wood and well supplied with water.

A Committee, in conjunction with the Managers, is entrusted with the charge of erecting the requisite buildings as soon as practicable. And it appears by the report of this Committee, that such progress has been made in procuring materials and engaging workmen, that the house will probably be carried up and roofed, in the early part of the ensuing autumn.

A view of the proposed building is prefixed to the present publication. The unavoidable extension of the front, arises from the necessity of affording comfort and convenience to the patients, by procuring a free admission of light and air. This important consideration will lead, in the first instance, to more expense, but we do not doubt will be fully counterbalanced by the advantages resulting from it.

A list of Contributors, and a statement of the amount of Contributions and Donations, as far as they have been ascertained, is subjoined.

Although the subscriptions already made afford a satisfactory evidence of the interest generally taken in this Institution, yet we look forward with a degree of confidence, in the continued liberality of Friends, to assist in carrying on and completing the intended design. Our Treasurer, John Hallowell, of Philadelphia, and the Agents of the Monthly Meetings, will receive the subscriptions and donations of Meetings and individuals: and the following form of a legacy is recommended to those who may be inclined to make bequests, by will.

FORM OF LEGACY.

I give and bequeath to A. B. and B. C. in trust for the use of an Institution near Philadelphia, known by the name of " The Contributors to the Asylum, for the relief of Persons deprived of the use of their Reason," the sum of

to be paid by the said Trustees to the Treasurer, for the time being, of the said Institution.

MONTHLY MEETINGS THAT HAVE SUBSCRIBED TO THE ASYLUM.

Philadelphia Monthly Meeting,	Samuel Betts,
Ditto, for the Northern District,	Joseph Scatt...
Ditto, for the Southern District,	William E...
Radnor,	Joseph Ge...
Exeter,	Thomas L...
Abington,	John L...
Byberry,	Ezra Townsend,
Horsham,	Giles Mitchell,
Gwynnedd,	
Solebury,	Oliver Paxson,
Wrightstown,	John Warner, Jr

Middletown,	Wm. Richardson, jr.
Falls,	John Brown.
Chester,	Francis Wisely.
Darby,	Edward Garrigues.
Goshen,	Jonas Preston.
Concord,	William Trimble.
Wilmington,	Evan Lewis.
Uwchlan,	Isaiah Kirk.
Kennet,	Edward Temple.
London Grove,	Joseph Pennock.
Fallowfield,	Isaac Pennock.
New Garden,	Enoch Lewis.
Duck Creek,	Daniel Cowgill.
Evesham,	Joseph Gardiner.
Haddonfield,	Joseph Kaighn.
Chester, N. Jersey,	John Collins.
Woodberry,	Paul Cooper.
Pilesgrove,	David Tatum.
Salem,	William F. Miller.
Maurice River,	Isaac Townsend.

CONTRIBUTORS TO THE ASYLUM.

Charles Allen*	Isaac Bonsall.
Joshua Ash.	Samuel Bettle.
William Abbott.	Clement Biddle, jr.
Joel Atkinson.	Titus Bennett.
John B. Ackley.	John Biddle.
Samuel Austin.	Philip S. Bunting.
Andrew Ashton.	Joseph Bacon.
	William Brown.
	Thomas Barnes.
	Jacob Ballanger.

* The Persons whose residence is not particularly desig-
nated, live within the limits of the Philadelphia Monthly
Meetings.

Edward Bonsall.
Henry Bowman, *Radnor Monthly Meeting.*
John F. Bunting, *Darby.*
Joseph Bassett, *Salem.*
John Bishop.

John Cooke.
Caleb Cresson, jr.
John E. Cresson.
James Cresson.
John H. Cresson.
Joseph Cresson.
Joseph Crukshank.
Caleb Carmalt.
Solomon W. Conrad.
Charles Comly.
Sharon Carter.
Angus Cameron.
Samuel Canby, jr.
Joseph Clark.
Samuel Canby, *Wilmington.*
William Carpenter, *Salem.*

Nathan Dunn.
Benjamin Davis.
Isaac Davis.
Evan Davis.

Ann Dawes.
Benedict Dorsey.
Sally N. Dickinson, *Wilmington.*

Jonathan Evans.
John Elliott.
Daniel Elliott.
Joshua Emlen.
Elizabeth Evans.
Anne Emlen.
Hannah Elliott.
Cadwalader Evans.
John C. Evans.
Joseph Evans.
David Evans, jr.
Jonas Eyre, *Chester.*
Samuel Emlen, *Burlington.*

William Folwell.
Charles C. French.
Jonathan Fell, jr.
Esther Fisher.
John Folwell, *Burlington.*

Elizabeth and Anna Guest.
Samuel P. Griffitts.

B

14

Philip Garrett.
Stacy Gillingham, *Abington.*
William Garrigues.
Edward Garrigues, *Darby,*
William Gibbons, *Wilmington.*
George W. Gibbons.
Samuel Griscom.

Robert Haydock.
William Haydock.
John Hallowell.
Eden Haydock.
Samuel Haydock.
Samuel E. Howell.
Benjamin Hornor.
Abraham Hilyard.
John G. Hoskins.
William Hallowell, jr.
Ephraim Haines.
Joseph Hartshorne.
John Hutchinson.
Richard Humphreys.
Israel Howell.
Hannah Hollingsworth.
Nathan Harper, *Abington.*
John Hunt, *Darby.*

Benjamin Johnson.

Jacob Johnson.
Josiah Johnson.
Benjamin Jones.
Jacob Justice.
Isaac C. Jones.
George Justice.
Joseph Justice.
Isaiah Jeanes.
David Jones.
Thomas C. James.
Jesse Jones, *Uwchlan:*
Rowland Jones, *Burlington.*

Emmor Kimber.
Thomas Kimber.
Thomas Kite.
Joseph Kirkbride.
George Knorr.
William Kinsey, *Abington.*

Samuel Lippincott.
Joshua Longstreth.
Isaac T. Longstreth.
Susanna Longstreth.
Samuel Longstreth.
Samuel N. Lewis.
Hannah Lewis.
Hannah Lewis, jr.
Mary Lewis.
Mary Lisle.

Margaret Lisle.
Thomas Loyd, jr.
John Lancaster.
Moses Lancaster.
Joseph Lea.
Jonathan Leedom.
Clement Laws.
Ludawick Laws.
Isaac Lawrence.
Thomas Lee, *Exeter*.
Martha Lancaster, *Falls*.
Thomas Lea, *Wilmington*.
Evan Lewis, *Wilmington*.
Ann Latimer, *Wilmington*.
Abraham Lower.

Ann Mifflin.
Richard M'Ilvaine, *Darby*.
Hugh M'Ilvaine, *Darby*.
John M'Ilvaine, *Chester*.
Josiah Miller, *Salem*.

Joseph P. Norris.
Thomas Norton.
Samuel Noble.
Martha Newbold.
John Newbold, *Chester*.

James Oldden, jr.

Thomas Martin.
James Martin.
Anne Mifflin.
Sarah Moore.
Israel Maule.
Gabriel Middleton.
Samuel Middleton.
Stephen Maxfield.
Isaac W. Morris.
John Morton.
Aaron Musgrave.
Thomas W. Morgan.
Lloyd Mifflin.
Phebe Morris.

Elliston Perot.
John Paul.
Joseph M. Paul.
Isaac Pearson.
Abraham L. Pennock.
Joseph Parrish.
Joseph Price.
Caleb Peirce.
Isaac Paxson.
William Paxson.
Thomas Parker.
Joseph Parker.

Edward Parker.
Sarah Pennock.
Abigail Physick.
Sarah Pemberton.
Henry Pemberton.
William Penrose.
William Price.
Thomas W. Pryor.
Isaac Peirce.
George Pryor.
Ann P. Paschall, *Darby.*
Levis Passmore, do.
Samuel Painter, *Concord.*
Robert L. Pitfield, *Burlington.*

Joseph Rotch.
Joseph Ridgway.
Nathaniel Richardson.
Joseph Richardson.
William R. Rodman.
Edward Randolph.
George F. Randolph.
Jacob Rodgers.
John Richardson.
George W. Robinson.
Rachel Richards.
Samuel Richards, S. S.

Thomas Scattergood.

Joseph Scattergood.
James Smith.
Abel Satterthwaite.
Isaac Smedley.
John D. Smith.
George R. Smith.
Joseph Sansom.
James Sellers.
Daniel Smith.
Stephen Simmons.
James Starr.
James Starr, jr.
Caleb Shreve.
Leonard Snowden.
Samuel Smith.
Joshua Sharpless, jr.
Mary Starr.
Richard Sermon.
James Sleeper.
John Simmons.
Charles E. Smith.
Samuel Story.
Samuel Smith.
Samuel Shinn.
Joseph Shoemaker.
Nathan Smith.
Edward Simmons, jr.
Stephen W. Smith.
Abraham Sharpless, *Concord.*
William Seal, *Wilmington.*
Samuel Swayne, *London-Grove.*
Samuel Shoemaker.
Stephen Smith.

Jonah Thompson.
John Tomlinson.
Benjamin Tucker.
Charles Townsend.
Joseph Thomas.
Jonathan Thomas.
James Truman.
Joseph Trotter.
Nathan Trotter.
Isaac Thomas.
John R. Thomas, *Uwchlan.*
Joseph Tatnall, *Wilmington.*

James Vaux.
Roberts Vaux.
Ann Vaux.

Nicholas Waln.
Thomas Wistar.
Caspar Wistar.
Barthlomew Wistar.
Sarah Wistar.
Hannah Wistar.
Edward Wilson.
George Williams.
Jonathan Willis.
William Wilson.
Joseph White.
Joseph Warner.
William Widdifield.

Hannah West.
Thomas Williams.
George Woolley.
Benjamin Williams.
Alexander Wilson.
John Ware.
Charles Wharton.
William Wharton.
Jacob S. Waln.
Nicholas Waln, jr.
Elizabeth Waln.
Phebe Waln.
Reed Williams.
Jesse Waterman.
Samuel West, *Chester.*
William Wright, *Sadsbury.*
Thomas Webster, *Abington.*
Jesse Walton, *do.*
Joel Woolman, *do.*
Isaac Whitelock, *do.*
Yeamans Gillingham, *do.*
Nathan Shoemaker, *do.*
John Wistar, *Salem.*

Ellis Yarnall.
Nathan Yarnall.
Benjamin H. Yarnall.
William Yardley.

Henry M. Zollickoffer.

CONTRIBUTIONS AND DONATIONS.

The Treasurer has received,
In contributions from Monthly
Meetings $5,995 75
   In contributions from members of
the Institution   17,040 00
   Donations from individuals   1,135 00

           Amount.   24,170 75

The following sums of money
have been paid by the Treasurer.
   For fifty-two acres of
ground,   6,764 06
   On account of the
building, &c.   2,041 04
   Balance remaining in
the Treasurer's hands,
Third Month, 12th, 1814, 15,365 65
                  24,170 75

From the estimates already made, it appears
that a considerable sum of money will be wanted,
in addition to the balance on hand, to complete the
proposed establishment. The necessity of ren-
dering the building secure from fire, will increase
the expense ; and we trust that these considerations will induce friends to be liberal in their subscriptions.

An abridged account of the proceedings of
Friends relative to the Retreat near York, in
England, is added, in order to convey correct information of the nature of the proposed establishment, the views of both institutions being
nearly the same.

DESCRIPTION

OF

THE RETREAT.

AN INSTITUTION NEAR YORK,

FOR INSANE PERSONS

OF THE

SOCIETY OF FRIENDS

ABRIDGED FROM THE ACCOUNT PUBLISHED.

BY SAMUEL TUKE.

PREFACE.

THE Establishment which is described in the following pages, though on a small scale, has so far met the approbation of many judicious persons, who have had an opportunity of minutely inspecting its internal economy and management, that I have been induced to attempt such a representation, as it is hoped will be useful to those who are engaged in similar institutions.

Contemplating the loss of reason as preeminent in the catalogue of human afflictions; and believing that the experience of the Retreat throws some light on the means of its mitigation, and also that it has demonstrated, beyond all contradiction, the superior efficacy, both in respect of cure and security, of a mild system of treatment in all cases of mental disorder, an account of that experience has long appeared to me, due to the public.

If it should be thought to afford satisfactory evidence in favour of a more mild system of treatment, than has been generally adopted; if it should also prove, which I flatter myself it will, the practicability of introducing such a system into establishments for the insane poor, whose situation has in general been too pitiable for words to describe, I shall esteem myself peculiarly happy in this publication.

The interests of humanity and science, alike call upon us to communicate freely the discoveries we make, or the failures which happen to us, in a pursuit so intimately connected with the happiness of our species.

I hope that my partiality for the establishment which I have endeavoured to describe, and my wish to present its objects and regulations to the public eye, have not induced me to deviate from that candour and sobriety of representation, which the reader has a right to expect. I am not conscious of such a deviation : but I well know that strong attachments, unless carefully guarded, are apt to impose upon our judgment. That this, however, has not been the case in the present instance, I am encouraged to believe, from the very favourable and commendatory characters, which have been given of the Institution, by several well informed and impartial persons, by whom it has been visited, and minutely examined.*

* It may be proper to observe, that, though the patients are never exhibited to gratify the curiosity

To support the statements given in this work of the modes of treatment at the Retreat, a few respectable testimonies in its favour are given in an Appendix. I am, however, far from imagining that this Asylum is a perfect model for others, either in regard to construction or management. If several improvements have been successfully introduced, it is probable that many others remain unattempted.

of visitors, yet professional persons, or those peculiarly interested in the subject, are permitted at all seasonable hours, to visit *every part* of the establishment. It would be well if this plan were generally adopted in other institutions of this nature, as the uncertainty of visitors arriving would be some check upon neglect, or improper conduct.

It may also be proper to state, that several persons about to engage in the superintendence of similar establishments, have made a temporary residence in York, and have been permitted by the Committee of the Retreat to observe daily the economy of the house, and the mode of managing the patients.

DESCRIPTION

OF

THE RETREAT, &c.

HISTORICAL ACCOUNT.

THE origin of the Institution which forms
the subject of the following pages, has much the
appearance of accident. In the year 1791, a female, of the Society of Friends, was placed at
an establishment for insane persons, in the vicini-
ty of the city of York: and her family, residing
at a considerable distance, requested some of
their acquaintance in the city to visit her. The
visits of these Friends were refused, on the
ground of the patient not being in a suitable state
to be seen by strangers: and, in a few weeks
after her admission, death put a period to her
sufferings.

The circumstance was affecting, and naturally
excited reflections on the situation of insane persons, and on the probable improvements which
might be adopted in establishments of this nature.
In particular, it was conceived that peculiar advantage would be derived to the Society of
Friends, by having an Institution of this kind
under their own care, in which a milder and

c

more appropriate system of treatment, than that
usually practised, might be adopted; and where
during lucid intervals, or the state of convalescence, the patient might enjoy the society of
those who were of similar habits and opinions.
It was thought, very justly, that the indiscriminate mixture, which must occur in large public
establisments, of persons of opposite religious
sentiments and practices; of the profligate and
the virtuous; the profane and the serious; was
calculated to check the progress of returning reason, and to fix, still deeper, the melancholy and
misanthropic train of ideas, which, in some des-
criptions of insanity, impresses the mind. It
was believed also, that the general treatment of
insane persons was, too frequently, calculated to
depress and degrade, rather than to awaken the
slumbering reason, or correct its wild hallucinations.

In one of the conversations to which the circumstance before-mentioned gave rise, the propriety of attempting to form an Establishment
for persons of our own Society, was suggested to
William Tuke, whose feelings were already
much interested in the subject, and whose persevering mind rendered him peculiarly eligible to
promote such an undertaking. After mature reflection, and several consultations with his most
intimate friends* on the subject, he was decidedly of opinion, that an Establishment for the
insane of our own Society, of every class in regard to property, was both eligible and highly de-

---

* Among the most early and strenuous friends of this
Establishment, I wish to particularize the name of the excellent Lindley Murray; to whose steady endeavours, for
promoting its welfare, the institution is much indebted.

sirable. It was necessary to excite a general interest in the Society on the subject. He therefore, after the close of the Quarterly Meeting at York, in the Third Month, 1792, requested Friends to allow him to introduce to them a subject, connected with the welfare of the Society. He then stated the views which he, and those whom he had consulted, had taken of this subject; the circumstance which had given rise to their interest respecting it, and the conviction which had resulted in their minds, in favour of an Institution under the government of Friends, for the care and accommodation of their own Members, labouring under that most afflictive dispensation—the loss of reason.

Few objections were then made, and several persons appeared to be impressed with the importance of the subject, and the propriety of the proposed measure. The friends with whom the proposal originated, were requested to prepare the outline of a plan, for the consideration of those who might attend the next Quarterly Meeting. Several objections, however, on a variety of grounds, soon afterward appeared. Many Friends were acquainted with but few, if any, objects for such an Establishment; and they seemed to forget that there might probably be many cases with which they were not acquainted. Some were not sensible that any improvement could be made in the treatment of the insane; supposing that the privations, and severe treatment, to which they were generally exposed, were necessary in their unhappy situation; and others, seemed rather averse to the concentration of the instances of this disease amongst us.

It was not, however, at all surprising that considerable diversity of opinion, should prevail upon a subject which was entirely new, and foreign to the general inquiries of those to whom it was proposed; and we must not forget that there was a respectable number, who duly appreciated the advantages likely to accrue to the Society from the proposed Establishment, and who cordially engaged in the promotion of the design. To these persons, and to the steady exertions of its chief promoter, whose mind was not to be deterred by ordinary difficulties, the Society of Friends may justly be said to owe the advantages it derives from this admirable Institution.

Some have thought that accommodations for so many as thirty patients, should not have been aimed at: But it is obvious, that the quantity of ground for exercise, ought not to be much, if any, less for fifteen than for thirty; that kitchens, parlours, and almost all parts of the building, except the number of patients' rooms, ought to be nearly the same; and that it would make little difference with respect to Physicians and domestic Managers: so that to accommodate the proposed number, would not only lessen the expense of each patient, but extend the benefits of the Institution to Friends at a greater distance.

It hath been said, that there are already many public Institutions of the kind, which render this unnecessary. But it is evident, besides what has been remarked on this head, in the former publication, that several peculiar and important advantages, will accrue from an Institution confined to ourselves. For as the disorder is a mental one, and people of regular conduct, and even religiously disposed minds, are not exempt from it, their confinement amongst persons in all respects strangers, and their promiscuous exposure to such company as is mostly found in public Institutions of this kind, must be peculiarly disgusting, and consequently augment their disorder. Nor is this idea merely chimerical; for it is well known, that the situation of divers Members of our Society, hath from this cause, been unspeakably distressing. A circumstance which, it needs no arguments to prove, must greatly retard, if not totally prevent their cure.

Friends who think the object worthy their attention, may be encouraged to promote it, not only on a principle of charity to the poor, but even of compassion to those in easy and affluent circumstances; who will doubtless think themselves benefited, though they may pay amply for it. Those who have embarked in this undertaking, have not been influenced by interested views, nor are they requesting or desiring any favours for themselves. A malady, in many instances, the most deplorable that human nature is subject to, hath excited their sympathy and attention; and they invite such Friends as approve of their design, to co-operate with them in an Establishment, which hath for its object, the mitigation of misery, and the restoration of those, who are lost to civil and religious society: in the prosecution whereof, they humbly rely on the favour of HIM, whose tender mercies are over all his works.

" In the short time that this Institution has been established, there has appeared abundant cause to convince us of the necessity there was for it; for a considerable disadvantage not only seems to have been sustained, in many cases, from unskilful private confinement; but there has also been particular occasion to observe the great loss, which individuals of our Society have sustained, by being put under the care of those, who are not only strangers to our principles, but by whom they are frequently mixed with other patients, who may indulge themselves in ill language, and other exceptionable practices. This often seems to leave an unprofitable effect upon the patients' minds, after they are restored to the use of their reason, alienating from those religious attachments which they had before experienced; and, sometimes, even corrupting them with vicious habits, to which they had been strangers.

In describing the particular benefits of this undertaking, it seems proper to mention that of occasionally using the patients to such employment, as may be suitable and proper for them, in order to relieve the languor of idleness, and prevent the indulgence of gloomy sensations. The privilege of attending religious meetings, when they are fit for it, and of having occasionally the visits of suitable Friends at the house, may be justly esteemed of no inconsiderable importance. These considerations, added to those which have already been mentioned, and that of the frequent attendance of Women Friends appointed every month, by a Committee which meets in the house, appear to give this Institution peculiar advantages, in the view of Friends; and to warrant the promoters of it in expecting the support and encouragement of the Society.

Experience has this year abundantly convinced us, of the advantage to be derived from an

early attention to persons afflicted with disorders
of the mind.

This consideration will, we hope, encourage
the friends of those who are, or may be afflicted
with this malady, to remove them early, and
place them under proper care and treatment.

DESCRIPTION AND APPROPRIATION OF THE GROUNDS AND HOUSE.

THE Retreat is situate on an eminence, at
the distance of about half a mile from the eastern gate of the city of York. It commands a
very delightful prospect, extending, on the south,
as far as the eye can reach, over a wooded, fertile plain; and terminating on the north and east,
by the Hambleton Hills and the Wolds; which
are seen, in some places, at the distance of about
twenty-five miles.

The situation combines nearly all the circumstances, which are usually considered favourable
to longevity; and the almost uniform health of
the family, has confirmed the general observations on this subject.

In the erection of the building, economy and
convenience have been chiefly consulted.

There are eleven acres of land belonging to
the Institution. This little farm is chiefly occupied in the growth of potatoes, and the support of the cows, which supply the family with
milk and butter.

The garden is on the north side of the house,
and contains about one acre. This furnishes abundance of fruit and vegetables. It also
affords an agreeable place for recreation and

employment, to many of the patients; being divided by gravel-walks, interspersed with shrubs and flowers, and sheltered from the intrusive eye of the passenger, by a narrow plantation and shrubbery.

On the south side of the house, are the courts for the different classes of patients. The circular wall which encloses the male and female patients' courts, are about eight feet high; but as the ground declines from the house, their apparent height is not so great; and the view from them of the country is consequently not so much obstructed, as it would be if the ground was level. I cannot, however, forbear observing, that the courts appear to be too small, and to admit of too little variety, to invite the patient to take exercise. The boundary of his excursion is always before his eye; which must have a gloomy effect on the already depressed mind. This might be considered as a serious defect, if it was not generally compensated, by taking such patients as are suitable, into the garden; and by frequent excursions into the city or the surrounding country, and into the fields of the Institution. One of these is surrounded by a walk, interspersed with trees and shrubs.

The superintendent has also endeavoured to furnish a source of amusement, to those patients whose walks are necessarily more circumscribed, by supplying each of the courts with a number of animals; such as rabbits, sea-gulls, hawks, and poultry. These creatures are generally very familiar with the patients: and it is believed that they are not only the means of innocent pleasure; but that the intercourse with them, sometimes tends to awaken the social and benevolent feelings.

An apartment is used, when necessary, for the entire seclusion of a violent patient. It is furnished with a bed, securely fastened to the ground. Light is, in great measure, but not entirely excluded; and care is taken to have the room properly ventilated.

This room also affords an opportunity of temporary confinement, by way of punishment, for any very offensive acts, which it is thought the patient had the power to restrain; but this very rarely occurs; and I am happy to say, the apartment is frequently unoccupied; or in other words, there is not, on an average, from any cause, one male patient in a state of seclusion during the day.

The attention which is due to the comfort of the insane, and the degree in which it is compatible with their security, appear to have been, till very recently, objects of little general consideration. It is not, therefore, to be supposed, that the Retreat, which has now been erected seventeen years, and which was originally intended for only thirty patients, should be a perfect model for establishments of this kind; though every care was exercised in its first construction. Indeed, it is hardly probable, as the class of persons, in different establishments, must be various, that the arrangements in any one, can be precisely followed in another.

The promoters of this Institution, as they observed in one of their early Reports, could not be supposed to be superior to those disadvantages, to which the want of experience naturally exposed them. When it is also considered, that they were unable to form any probable opinion, of the proportions of the different class of patients; and that the number has, unhappily, much exceeded their expectations, it will not

surprising, that the building has several imper--
fections, but rather that it possesses so many advantages.

It has been already observed, that the aspect
of a place of confinement is prevented, by the
substitution of cast iron window frames for the
bars, which, in similar places, usually guarded
the avenues of light. This contrivance unites
the advantages of security, neatness, and durabi-
lity. There are not in this house any cells under ground. All the rooms, except three which
derive their light from an adjoining gallery, have
glass windows. Iron bars and shutters, are too
often substituted for glazed windows, in rooms
appropriated to the insane. The obvious consequence is, that the air, however cold, cannot be
kept out of the apartment, without the entire ex-
clusion of light.

*One circumstance, which I much regret, in the
construction of this building, is, that there are
rooms on both sides of the galleries; for, though
a large portion of light is admitted, by the window at each extremity of the building, yet, the
galleries on the ground floor, at least, are rather
gloomy.*

*I observe with pleasure, in a very ingenious
account and plan of a new asylum at Glasgow*
that the galleries have rooms on one side, and
windows on the other. This cannot fail to give
an air of cheerfulness, highly desirable in such
establishments.*

---

* " Remarks on the Construction of Public Hospitals," by
Wm. Stark, Esq. architect. This work, as well as " Observations on the Treatment of Lunatics," by Robert Reid,
Esq. architect, deserves the attention of those who are engaged in such undertakings.

Many errors in the construction, as well as in the management of asylums for the insane, appear to arise from excessive attention to *safety*. People, in general, have the most erroneous notions of the constantly outrageous behaviour, or malicious dispositions, of deranged persons; and it has, in too many instances, been found convenient to encourage these false sentiments, to apologize for the treatment of the unhappy sufferers, or admit the vicious neglect of their attendants.*

In the construction of such places, cure and comfort ought to be as much considered, as security; and, I have no hesitation in declaring, that a system which, by limiting the power of the attendant, obliges him not to neglect his duty, and makes it his interest to obtain the good opinion of those under his care, provides more effectually for the safety of the keeper, as well as of the patient, than all " the apparatus of chains, darkness, and anodynes."

MEDICAL TREATMENT.

UNDER the head " Medical treatment," as practised in the Retreat, some may possible inquire, what are the means employed in mortifications, arising from cold and confinement? " a calamity, which," says a writer before alluded to,

* I once accidentally visited a house for insane persons, in which security was made a *primary* object. Here I saw three of the keepers, in the middle of the day, earnestly employed in—*playing at cards !*

" frequently happens to the helpless insane, and to bed-ridden patients; as my attendance in a large work-house, in private mad-houses, and Bethlem Hospital, can amply testify."*

Haslam also observes, that the patients in Bethlem Hospital, " are particularly subject to mortifications of the feet; and this fact is so well established from former accidents, that there is an express order of the house, that every patient, under strict confinement, shall have his feet examined every morning and evening in the cold weather, by the keeper, and also have them constantly wrapped in flannel; and those who are permitted to go about, are always to be found as near to the fire as they can get, during the winter season."†

Dr. Pinel also confesses, that " seldom has a whole year elapsed, during which no fatal accident has taken place, in the Hospital de Bicetre, (in France,) from the action of cold upon the extremities."

Happily, in the Institution I am now describing, this calamity is hardly known; and no instance of mortification has occurred, in which it has been, in any degree connected with cold or confinement. Indeed the patients are never found to require such a degree of restraint, as to prevent the use of considerable exercise, or to render it at all necessary to keep their feet wrapped in flannel.

It will be proper here to observe, that the experience of the Retreat, fully confirms the opinion of several respectable modern writers, that

* Crowther, p. 61.
† Observations on Madness, p. 84.

maniacs are by no means exempted from the
common effects of cold ; and it is to be hoped,
for the sake of humanity, that the opposite opinion, alike barbarous and absurd, will be entirely exploded. The apothecary to Bethlem Hospital, after stating that the patients are not exempt from the usual effects of severe cold, observes very justly : " from the great degree of
insensibility which prevails, in some states of
madness, a degree of cold would scarcely be felt
by such persons, which would create uneasiness
in those of sound mind but experience has
shown that they suffer equally from severity of
weather. When the mind is particularly engaged on any subject, external circumstances affect
us less, than when unoccupied. Every one must
recollect, that in following up a favourite pursuit, his fire has burned out without his being
sensible of the alteration of temperature ; but
when the performance has been finished, or he
has become indifferent to it from fatigue, he then
becomes sensible to cold, which he had not experienced before."

The supporters of this opinion, also generally
observe, that insane persons commonly endure
hunger without injury. The latter sentiment is
no less at variance with the experience of the
Retreat, than the former. Some of the patients,
more especially the melancholics and convalescents, besides their four usual meals in the day,
require the intermediate refreshment of biscuit,
with a glass of wine or porter ; and attention of
this kind is considered almost essential to the
recovery of many patients.

"General propositions," says Dr. Pinel, "have been too often advanced in regard to the capacity of maniacs to bear extreme hunger with impunity. I have known several, who were voracious to a great degree, and who languished, even to fainting, from want, or deficiency of nourishment. It is said of an Asylum at Naples, that a low spare diet is a fundamental principle of the Institution. It would be difficult to trace the origin of so singular a prejudice. Unhappy experience, which I acquired during seasons of scarcity, has most thoroughly convinced me, that insufficiency of food, when it does not altogether extinguish the vital principle, is not a little calculated to exasperate and prolong the disease."*

I would not have dwelt so long upon these mistaken opinions, if they had not furnished a specious pretext for much practical barbarity; and I am, therefore, anxious to see them ranked with the marvellous stories of the Phœnix and the Salamander.

Where various means are employed, it is difficult to say which is the operative one; but, whatever may be the means used, there is great reason to believe that a clear dry air, which the situation of the Retreat affords in an eminent degree, will facilitate their operation, and be favourable to the recovery of insane persons. To reason again from analogy; the general effect of fine air upon the animal spirits, would induce us to expect especial benefit from it, in cases of mental depression; and to pay all due respect to the physician, who,

* Dr. Davis's translation of "Pinel's Treatise on Insanity," p. 31.

"Gives melancholy up to Nature's care,
And sends the patient into purer air."

Several instances have occurred, in which melancholy patients have been very much improved by their journey to the Retreat; and it is the
decided opinion of the manager of this Institution, that, in such cases, close confinement is, of
all things, the most detrimental.

MORAL TREATMENT.

WHATEVER theory we maintain in regard
to the remote causes of insanity, we must consider moral treatment, or management, of very
high importance.

If we adopt the opinion, that the disease origi-
nates in the mind, applications made immediately to it, are obviously the most natural; and the
most likely to be attended with success. If, on
the contrary, we conceive that mind is incapable
of injury or destruction, and that, in all cases of
apparent mental derangement, some bodily disease, though unseen and unknown, really exists,
we shall still readily admit, from the reciprocal
action of the two parts of our system upon each
other, that the greatest attention is necessary, to
whatever is calculated to affect the mind.

It is a matter of no small difficulty, to convey
more than the general principles which influence
the conduct of those, who have the management of the insane. It is unhappily, in great
measure true, that "the address which is acquired by experience, and constant intercourse

with maniacs, cannot be communicated: it may
be learned; but it must perish with its posses-
sors." It appears, however, to me, that a free
detail of different modes of management, can
hardly fail to increase our stock of correct general principles, on this important subject.

Insane persons generally possess a degree of
control over their wayward propensities. Their
intellectual, active, and moral powers, are usually rather perverted than obliterated; and it
happens, not unfrequently, that one faculty
only is affected. The disorder is sometimes
still more partial, and can only be detected by
erroneous views, on one particular subject. On
all others, the mind appears to retain its wonted
correctness.

The same *partial* perversion, is found to obtain in this disease with regard to the affections.
Though it frequently happens, that indifference
or disgust towards the tenderest connexions, is
an early and distressing symptom of insanity;
when,

> ———————— " forgotten quite,
> All former scenes of dear delight,
> Connubial love, parental joy;
> No sympathies like these his soul employ;"

yet the existence of the benevolent affections, is
often strongly evidenced, by the patients' attachment to those who have the immediate care of
them, and who treat them with judgment and
humanity. The apothecary to Bethlem Hospital says,* " I can truly declare, that by gen-
tleness of manner, and kindness of treatment, I
have seldom failed to obtain the confidence, and
conciliate the esteem, of insane persons; and

* Observations, p. 293.

have succeeded by these means in procuring from them respect and obedience." The superintendents of the Retreat give precisely the same evidence; and I firmly believe, that a large majority of the instances, in which the malevolent dispositions are peculiarly apparent, and are considered as characterizing the disorder, may readily be traced to secondary causes; arising from the peculiar circumstances of the patient, or from the mode of management.

A patient confined at home, feels naturally a degree of resentment, when those whom he has been accustomed to command, refuse to obey his orders, or attempt to restrain him. We may also, I conceive, in part, attribute to similar secondary causes, that apparent absence of the social affections, and that sad indifference to the accustomed sources of domestic pleasure, of which we have just been speaking. The unhappy maniac is frequently unconscious of his own disease. He is unable to account for the change in the conduct of his wife, his children, and his surrounding friends. They appear to him cruel, disobedient, and ungrateful. His disease aggravates their conduct in his view, and leads him to numerous unfounded suspicions. Hence, the estrangement of his affections may frequently be the natural consequence, of either the proper and necessary, or of the mistaken conduct of his friends towards him.

In such cases, the judicious kindness of others appears generally to excite the gratitude and affection of the patient. Even in those deplorable instances where the ingenious humanity of the superintendent fails to conciliate, and the jaundice-like disease changes the very aspect of nature, and represents all mankind as the leagued enemies of the patient, the existence of the social affections, has often been strikingly evidenced, by attachment to some of the inferior animals.

There are, undoubtedly, cases in which the disorder is chiefly marked by a mischievous malevolent disposition; but of these, very few have occurred at the Retreat. There have, however, been many patients, in whom these dispositions have been occasionally conspicuous, or easily excited by improper treatment.

If the preceding sketch is correct, it would not, I apprehend, be difficult to infer theoretically, the general principles of moral treatment and management; but I have happily little occasion for theory, since my province is to relate, not only what ought to be done, but also what, in most instances, is actually performed.

The moral treatment of the insane, seems to divide itself into three parts; and under these, the practices of the Retreat may be arranged. We shall therefore inquire,

I. By what means the power of the patient to control the disorder, is strengthened and assisted.

II. What modes of coercion are employed, when restraint is absolutely necessary.

III. By what means the general comfort of the insane is promoted.

OF THE MEANS OF ASSISTING THE PATIENT TO CONTROL HIMSELF.

WE have already observed, that most insane persons have a considerable degree of self command; and that the employment and cultivation of this remaining power, is found to be attended with the most salutary effects. Though many cannot be made sensible of the irrationality of their conduct or opinions; yet they are generally aware of those particulars, for which the world considers them proper objects of confinement. Thus it frequently happens, in the Institution we are describing, that a patient, on his first introduction, will conceal all marks of mental aberration. Instances have occurred, in which the struggle has been so successful, that persons, who, on undoubted authority, have been declared to be unmanageable at home; and to have shown very striking marks of insanity; have not, for a very considerable time, exhibited sufficient symptoms of the disorder, to enable the physician to declare them, *non compos mentis*. Doubtless the idea that their early liberation, for which most are anxious, and their treatment during their confinement, will depend, in great measure, on their conduct, has a tendency to produce this salutary restraint, upon their wayward propensities. Hence, also, the idea seems to have arisen, that madness in all its forms, is capable of entire control, by a sufficient excitement of the principle of fear. This speculative opinion, though every day's experience decidedly contradicts it, is the best apology which can be made for the barbarous practices that have often prevailed in the treatment of the insane.

The principle of fear, which is rarely decreased by insanity, is considered as of great importance in the management of the patients. But it is not allowed to be excited, beyond that degree which naturally arises from the necessary regu-

lations of the family. Neither chains nor corporal punishments are tolerated, on any pretext,
in this establishment. The patients, therefore,
cannot be threatened with these severities; yet,
in all houses established for the reception of the
insane, the general comfort of the patients ought
to be considered; and those who are violent,
require to be separated from the more tranquil.
and to be prevented, by some means, from offensive conduct, towards their fellow-sufferers.
Hence, the patients are arranged into classes, as much as may be, according to the degree
in which they approach to rational or orderly
conduct.

They quickly perceive, or if not, they are informed on the first occasion, that their treatment
depends, in great measure, upon their conduct.
Coercion thus flowing as a sort of necessary consequence, and being executed in a manner which
marks the reluctance of the attendant, it seldom
exasperates the violence of the patient, or produces that feverish and sometimes furious irritability, in which the maniacal character is completely
developed; and under which all power of self-
control is utterly lost.

There cannot be a doubt that the principle of
fear, in the human mind, when moderately and
judiciously excited, as it is by the operation of
just and equal laws, has a salutary effect upon
society. It is a principle also of great use in the
education of children, whose imperfect knowledge and judgment, occasion them to be less
influenced by other motives. But where fear is
too much excited, and where it becomes the
chief motive of action, it certainly tends to con-

tract the understanding, to weaken the benevolent affections, and to debase the mind. As the
poet of liberty has well sung,

———————————" All constraint,
Except what wisdom lays on evil man,
Is evil; hurts the faculties, impedes
Their progress in the road of science, blinds
The eye-sight of discovery; and begets,
In those that suffer it, a sordid mind,
Bestial, a meagre intellect, unfit
To be the tenant of man's noble form."
COWPER'S TASK, BOOK V.

It is therefore wise to excite, as much as possible, the operation of superior motives; and
fear ought only to be induced, when a *necessary*
object cannot otherwise be obtained. If this is
the true scale of estimating the degree in which
this principle is, in general, to be employed, it
is found, at the Retreat, equally applicable to the
insane.

That the continual or frequent excitement of
the sensations of fear, should " bid melancholy
cease to mourn," is an idea too obviously absurd
in theory, to require the refutation of experience.
There has, however, unhappily been too much
experience on this subject; and hence we may
perhaps, in great degree, explain, why melancholy has been considered so much less susceptible
of cure than mania. To the mild system of
treatment adopted at the Retreat, I have no
doubt we may partly attribute, the happy recovery of so large a portion of melancholy patients.

Is then the violent excitement of the principle of fear, better adapted to enable the maniac
to control his wanderings, and to suppress his

emotions? Is it not well known, that the passions of many maniacs, are extremely irritable? and when once excited, are not all moral means to subdue them, as ineffectual as the attempt would be to quench, by artificial means, the fires of Etna?

If it be true, that oppression makes a *wise* man mad, is it to be supposed that stripes, and insults, and injuries, for which the receiver knows no cause, are calculated to make a *madman* wise? or would they not exasperate his disease, and excite his resentment? May we not hence most clearly perceive, why furious mania is almost a stranger in the Retreat? why all the patients wear clothes, and are generally induced to adopt orderly habits?

The superintendent of this Institution is fully of opinion, that a state of furious mania is very often excited by the mode of management. Of this opinion, a striking illustration occurred in this Institution, some years ago. A patient, of rather a vindictive and self-important character, who had previously conducted himself with tolerable propriety, one day, climbed up against a window, which overlooked the court where he was confined, and amused himself by contemplating the interior of the room. An attendant, who had not been long in office, perceiving his situation, ran hastily towards him, and, without preamble, drew him to the ground. The patient was highly incensed; a scuffle immediately ensued, in which he succeeded in throwing his antagonist; and had not the loud vociferations of this attendant alarmed the family, it is probable that he would have paid for his rash conduct, by the loss of his life. The furious state of the patient's mind did not continue long; but. after this circumstance, he was more vindictive and violent.

In some instances, the superintendent has known furious mania temporarily induced, by the privations necessary on a relapse, after a considerable lucid interval, during which the patient had enjoyed many privileges, that were incompatible with his disordered state. Here we may suggest the expediency, where it is possible, of employing such of the attendants to control the patient during his paroxyms, as had little intercourse with him in his lucid interval. Instances of furious mania have been, however, very rare ; but a considerable number of patients have been admitted, who were reported to have been so furiously insane, as to require constant coercion.

The evidence of attendants, who have been employed, previously to the admission of patients into the Retreat, is not considered a sufficient reason for any extraordinary restraint; and cases have occurred, in which persuasion and kind treatment, have superseded the necessity of any coercive means.

Some years ago, a man about thirty-four years of age, of almost Herculean size and figure, was brought to the house. He had been fettered several times before ; and so constantly during the present attack. had he been confined, that his clothes were contrived to be taken off and put on by means of strings, without removing his manacles. They were, however, taken off, when he entered the Retreat, and he was ushered into the apartment, where the superintendents were supping. He was calm; his attention appeared to be arrested by his new situation. He was desired to join in the repast, during which he behaved with tolerable propriety. After it was concluded, the superintendent conducted him to his apartment, and told him the circumstances on which his treatment would depend; that it was his anxious wish to make every inhabitant in the house, as comfortable as possible; and that he sincerely hoped the patient's conduct would render it unnecessary for him to have recourse to coercion. The maniac was sensible of the kindness of his treatment. He promised to restrain himself, and he so completely succeeded, that, during his stay, no coercive means were ever employed towards him. This case affords a striking example of the efficacy of mild treatment. The patient was frequently very vociferous, and threatened his attendants, who in their defence were very desirous of restraining him by the jacket. The superintendent, on these occasions, went to his apartment; and though the first sight of him seemed rather to increase the patient's irritation, yet after sitting some time quietly beside him, the violent excitement subsided, and he would listen with attention to the persuasions and arguments of his friendly visitor.

After such conversations, the patient was generally better for some days or a week; and in about four months he was discharged perfectly recovered.

Can it be doubted, that, in this case, the disease had been greatly exasperated by the mode of management? or that the subsequent kind treatment, had a great tendency to promote his recovery?

49

It may probably be urged, and I am very well aware of it, that there is a considerable class of patients, whose eccentricities may, in great measure, be controlled; and who may be kept in subjection and apparent orderly habits, by the strong excitement of the principle of fear. They may be made to obey their keepers, with the greatest promptitude; to rise, to sit, to stand, to walk, or run at their pleasure; though only expressed by a look. Such an obedience, and even the appearance of affection, we not unfrequently see in the poor animals who are exhibited to gratify our curiosity in natural history; but who can avoid reflecting, in observing such spectacles, that the readiness with which the savage tyger obeys his master, is the result of treatment at which humanity would shudder; and shall we propose by such means,

> " To calm the tumult of the breast,
> Which madness has too long possest;
> To chase away the fiend Despair,
> To clear the brow of gloomy Care;
> Bid pensive melancholy cease to mourn,
> Calm Reason reassume her seat;
> Each intellectual power return?"

If those who are friendly to what may be termed the terrific system of management, could prove, that, notwithstanding it may fix for life, the misery of a large majority of the melancholics; and drive many of the more irritable maniacs to fury or desperation; yet that it is still, in its operation upon a large scale, adapted to promote the cure of insanity, they would have some apology for its indiscriminate adoption. If, on the contrary, a statement of the proportion of cures in the Retreat, shall sufficiently prove

E

the superior efficacy of mild means, would not those, who are adopting an opposite line of treatment, do well to reflect on the awful responsibility which attaches to their conduct? Let us all constantly remember, that there is a Being, to whose eye darkness is light; who sees the inmost recesses of the dungeon, and who has declared, " For the sighing of the poor, and the crying of the needy, I will arise."

From the view we have now taken of the propriety of exciting fear, as a mean of promoting the cure of insanity, by enabling the patient to control himself, it will, perhaps, be almost superfluous to state as our opinion, that the idea, which has too generally obtained, of its being necessary to commence an acquaintance with lunatics, by an exhibition of strength, or an appearance of austerity, is utterly erroneous. The sentiment appears allied to that cruel system, probably dictated by indolence and timidity, which has so long prevailed, and unhappily still prevails, in many receptacles for the insane.

There is much analogy between the judicious treatment of children, and that of insane persons. Locke has observed, that " the great secret of education, lies in finding the way to keep the child's spirit easy, active, and free; and yet, at the same time, to restrain him from many things he has a mind to, and to draw him to things which are uneasy to him." It is highly desirable that the attendants on lunatics should possess this influence over their minds; but it will never be obtained by austerity and rigour; nor will assumed consequence, and airs of self-importance, be generally more successful.

Much familiarity with maniacal patients, on their first introduction to a new situation, is not thought, in general, to be adviseable. It might, in some instances, have a tendency to lessen that authority, which is, occasionally, necessary for the attendant to exert. There may also be a few cases in which a distant, and somewhat important manner, may be assumed with advantage; but, generally speaking, even with regard to the more violent and vociferous maniacs, a very different mode is found successful; and they are best approached with soft and mild persuasion. The superintendent assures me, that in these cases, he has found it peculiarly necessary to speak to th epatient in a kind, and somewhat low tone of voice. So true are the maxims of antiquity.

" A soft answer turneth away wrath."—SOLOMON.
———————— " Soft speech
" Is to distemper'd wrath, medicinal."—ÆSCHYLUS.

It must, however, be understood, that the persuasion, which is extended to the patients, is confined to those points which affect their liberty or comfort. No advantage has been found to arise from reasoning with them, on their particular hallucinations. One of the distinguishing marks of insanity, is a fixed false conception, which occasions an almost total incapacity of conviction. The attempt, therefore, to refute their notions, generally irritates them, and fixes the false perception more strongly on their minds. There have been a few instances, in which, by some striking evidence, the maniac has been driven from his favourite absurdity; but it has uniformly been succeeded by another equally irrational.

In regard to melancholics, conversation on the subject of their despondency, is found to be highly injudicious. The very opposite method is pursued. Every means is taken to seduce the mind from its favourite but unhappy musings, by bodily exercise, walks, conversations, reading, and other innocent recreations. The good effect of exercise, and of variety of object, has been very striking in several instances at this Institution. Some years ago, a patient much afflicted with melancholic and hypochondriacal symptoms, was admitted by his own request. He had walked from home, a distance of 200 miles, in company with a friend, and on his arrival, found much less inclination to converse on the absurd and melancholy views of his own state, than he had previously felt.

This patient was by trade a gardener, and the superintendent immediately perceived, from the effect of this journey, the propriety of keeping him employed. He led him into the garden, and conversed with him on the subject of horticulture; and soon found that the patient possessed very superior knowledge of pruning, and of the other departments of his art. He proposed several improvements in the management of the garden, which were adopted, and the gardener was desired to furnish him with full employment. He soon, however, showed a reluctance to regular exertion, and a considerable disposition to wandering, which had been one of the previous features of his complaint. The gardener was repeatedly charged to encourage him in labour, and to prevent his leaving the premises. But, unhappily, the superior abilities of the patient, had excited a jealousy in the gardener's mind, which made him dislike his assistance; and it may therefore be presumed, that he obeyed his instructions very imperfectly.

The poor man rambled several times from the grounds of the Institution; which, in his state of mind, excited considerable anxiety in the family. Of course it became necessary to confine him more within doors. He frequently, however, walked out; and the superintendant took many opportunities to attend him into the fields or garden, and to engage him for a time in steady manual labour. As his disorder had increased, it became difficult to induce him to exert himself; but even in this state, when he had been some time employed, he seemed to forget his distressing sensations and ideas, and would converse on general topics with great good sense.

In this truly pitiable case, the superintendant several times tried the efficacy of long walks, where the greatest variety and attraction of circumstances were presented; but neither these, nor the conversation which he introduced, were able to draw the patient so effectually from the " moods of his own mind," as regular persevering labour in the garden. It is not improbable, however, that the superior manner in which the patient was able to execute his work, produced a degree of self-complacency which had a salutary effect; and that, had his education enlarged his curiosity, and encouraged a taste and observation respecting the objects of nature and art, he might have derived much greater advantage, as many patients obviously do, from variety of conversation and scenery.

The circumstances of this patient did not allow him a separate attendant, and the engagements of the superintendent were too numerous and important, to permit him to devote to this case the time and attention which it seemed to require. He has frequently expressed to me, the strong feelings of regret, which were excited in his mind, by the unsuccessful treatment of this patient; the case certainly points out the great importance of exercise and labour, in the moral treatment of insanity, more especially in cases of melancholy.

This patient, after remaining several years in the house, died of an acute inflammation of the bowels. His situation for a considerable time previously to his death, was most deplorable, and has often reminded me of the affecting description, which our great poet gives of the state of our first father, after his expulsion from the happy seat of primeval innocence:

> ——————— " On the ground,
> Outstretch'd he lay, on the cold ground, and oft
> Curs'd his creation, death as oft accus'd
> Of tardy execution."

The female patients in the Retreat, are employed, as much as possible, in sewing, knitting, or domestic affairs; and several of the convalescents assist the attendants. Of all the modes by which the patients may be induced to restrain themselves, regular employment is perhaps the most generally efficacious; and those kinds of employment are doubtless to be preferred, both on a moral and physical account, which are accompanied by considerable bodily action; that are most agreeable to the patient, and which are most opposite to the illusions of his disease.

In an early part of this chapter, it is stated, that the patients are considered capable of rational and honourable inducement; and though we allowed *fear* a considerable place in the production of that restraint, which the patient generally exerts on his entrance into a new situation; yet the *desire of esteem* is considered, at the Retreat, as operating, in general, still more powerfully. This principle in the human mind, which doubtless influences, in a great degree, though often secretly, our general manners; and which operates with peculiar force on our introduction into a new circle of acquaintance, is found to have great influence, even over the conduct of the insane. Though it has obviously not been sufficiently powerful to enable them entirely to resist the strong irregular tendencies of their disease; yet when properly cultivated, it leads many to struggle to conceal and overcome their morbid propensities; and, at least, materially assists them in confining their deviations, within such bounds, as do not make them obnoxious to the family.

This struggle is highly beneficial to the patient, by strengthening his mind, and conducing to a salutary habit of self-restraint: an object which experience points out as of the greatest importance, in the cure of insanity by moral means.

That fear is not the only motive, which operates in producing *self-restraint* in the minds of maniacs, is evident from its being often exercised in the presence of strangers, who are merely passing through the house; and which, I presume, can only be accounted for, from that desire of esteem, which has been stated to be a powerful motive to conduct.

It is probably from encouraging the action of this principle, that so much advantage has been found in this Institution, for treating the patient as much in the manner of a rational being, as the state of his mind will possibly allow. The superintendent is particularly attentive to this point, in his conversation with the patients. He introduces such topics as he knows will most interest them; and which, at the same time, allows them to display their knowledge to the greatest advantage. If the patient is an agriculturist, he asks him questions relative to his art; and frequently consults him upon any occasion in which his knowledge may be useful. I have heard one of the worst patients in the house, who, previously to his indisposition, had been a considerable grazier, give very sensible directions for the treatment of a diseased cow.

These considerations are undoubtedly very material, as they regard the comfort of insane persons; but they are of far greater importance, as they relate to the cure of the disorder. The patient feeling himself of some consequence, is induced to support it by the exertion of his reason, and by restraining those dispositions, which, if indulged, would lessen the respectful treatment he receives; or lower his character in the eyes of his companions and attendants.

They who are unacquainted with the character of insane persons, are very apt to converse with them in a childish, or, which is worse, in a domineering manner; and hence it has been frequently remarked by the patients at the Retreat, that a stranger who had visited them, seemed to imagine they were children.

The natural tendency of such treatment is, to degrade the mind of the patient, and to make him indifferent to those moral feelings, which, under judicious direction and encouragement, are found capable, in no small degree, to strengthen the power of self-restraint; and which render the resort to coercion, in many cases, unnecessary. Even when it is absolutely requisite to employ coercion, if the patient promises to control himself on its removal, great confidence is generally placed upon his word. I have known patients, such is their sense of honour and moral obligation, under this kind of engagement, hold, for a long time, a successful struggle with the violent propensities of their disorder; and such attempts ought to be sedulously encouraged by the attendant.

Hitherto we have chiefly considered those modes of inducing the patient to control his disordered propensities, which arise from an application to the general powers of the mind; but considerable advantage may certainly be derived, in this part of moral management, from an acquaintance with the previous habits, manners, and prejudices of the individual. Nor must we forget to call to our aid, in endeavouring to promote self-restraint, the mild but powerful influence of the precepts of our holy religion. Where these have been strongly imbued in early life, they become little less than principles of our nature; and their restraining power is frequently felt, even under the delirious excitement of insanity. To encourage the influence of religious principles over the mind of the insane, is considered of great consequence, as a mean of cure. For this purpose, as well as for others, still more important, it is certainly right to promote in the patient, an attention to his accustomed modes of paying homage to his Maker.

Many patients attend the religious meetings of the Society, held in the city ; and most of them are assembled, on a first day afternoon ; at which time the superintendent reads to them several chapters in the Bible. A profound silence generally ensues ; during which, as well as at the time of reading, it is very gratifying to observe their orderly conduct, and the degree in which those, who are much disposed to action, restrain their different propensities.

In pursuing these desirable objects, let not tne inexperienced, but judicious attendant, expect too immediate effects from his endeavours, or be disheartened by occasional disappointment. Let him bear in mind, what the great Lord Bacon has admirably said, that " It is order, pursuit, sequence, and interchange of application, which is mighty in nature ; which, although it require more exact knowledge in prescribing, and more precise obedience in observing, yet is recompensed with the magnitude of effects."*

I am sensible that what is here stated, is but an imperfect view of the principles and modes, by which self-restraint is induced at the Retreat. To particularize all the principles of the mind, which may be usefully excited in promoting this salutary object, would be an enumeration of our intellectual powers and affections. I will only further observe upon this head, by way of general summary, that the attendant on the insane, ought sedulously to endeavour to gain

* Works, 8vo edition, vol. i. p. 125.

their confidence and esteem; to arrest their attention, and fix it on objects opposite to their illusions; to call into action, as much as possible, every remaining power and principle of the mind; and to remember that, in the wreck of the intellect, the affections not unfrequently survive.

OF THE MODES OF COERCION.

With regard to the second point, the necessity of coercion, I have no hesitation in saying, that it will diminish or increase, as the moral treatment of the patient is more or less judicious. We cannot, however, anticipate that the most enlightened and ingenious humanity, will ever be able entirely to supersede the necessity of personal restraint.

Coercion is considered, as the ingenious author of "Observations on Madness" says it should be, "only as a protecting and salutary restraint." The mode of it ought to be subject to the consideration of its effect on the mind of the insane. Some means of coercion have a obviously a greater tendency than others, to irritate or degrade the feelings. Hence, the use of chains has never been permitted in the treat. In the most violent states of mania, as the author just quoted observes, "the patient should be kept alone, in a dark* and quiet room, so that he may not be affected by the stimuli of light or sound; such abstraction more easily

---

* Our superintendent prefers a gloomy, to an entirely dark apartment.

ly disposing to sleep. As in this violent state, there is a strong propensity to associate ideas, it is particularly important to prevent the accession of such as might be transmitted through the medium of the senses."* The patients of this class, who are not disposed to injure themselves, are merely confined by the strait-waistcoat; and left to walk about the room, or lie down on the bed, at pleasure. But in those desperate cases of melancholy, attended with tædium vitæ, in which there is a strong determination to self-destruction, it becomes necessary to confine the patient, during the night, in a recumbent posture. For this purpose, the superintendent has invented a very simple apparatus, which answers all the purposes of security; and allows the patient to turn and otherwise change his posture in bed.

It has been suggested, that in cases of high mania, the violent excitement would be best reduced, by indulging it in the greatest practicable degree. The experience of the Retreat, leads to an opposite conclusion; viz. that such a degree of restraint as would not be materially painful, in a state of calmness, has a tendency to abate the paroxysm. The association between mental and bodily action, and the degree in which the latter is well known to excite the former, sufficiently illustrate the cause of this fact.

Except in the case of violent mania, which is far from being a frequent occurrence at the Retreat, coercion, when requisite, is considered as a necessary evil; that is, it is thought abstractedly to have a tendency to retard the cure

* The necessity for this mode of treatment is very rare at the Retreat.

by opposing the influence of the moral remedies employed. It is therefore used very sparingly : and the superintendent has often assured me, that he would rather run some risk, than have recourse to restraint, where it was not absolutely necessary; except in those cases where it was likely to have a salutary moral tendency.

I feel no small satisfaction in stating upon the authority of the superintendents, that during the last year, in which the number of patients has generally been sixty-four, there has not been occasion to seclude, on an average, two patients at one time. I am also able to state, that although it is occasionally necessary to restrain by the waistcoat, straps, or other means, several patients at one time; yet that the average number so restrained does not exceed four, including those who are secluded.

The safety of those who attend upon the Insane, is certainly an object of great importance; but it is worthy of inquiry whether it may not be attained, without materially interfering with another object—the recovery of the patient. It may also deserve inquiry, whether the extensive practice of coercion, which obtains in some Institutions, does not arise from erroneous views of the character of insane persons ; from indifference to their comfort ; or from having rendered coercion necessary by previous unkind treatment.

The power of judicious kindness over this unhappy class of society, is much greater than is generally imagined.

In no instances has this power been more strikingly displayed ; or exerted, with more beneficial effects, than in those deplorable cases in

F

which the patient refuses to take food. The kind persuasions and ingenious arts of the superintendents, have been singularly successful in overcoming this distressing symptom; and very few instances now occur in which it is necessary to employ violent means for supplying the patient with food.

Some patients who refuse to partake of the family-meals, are induced to eat by being taken into the larder, and there allowed to help themselves. Some are found willing to eat when food is left with them in their rooms, or when they can obtain it unobserved by their attendants. Others, whose determination is stronger, are frequently induced, by repeated persuasion, to take a small quantity of nutritious liquid; and it is equally true in these, as in general cases, that every breach of resolution weakens the power and disposition to resistance.

Sometimes, however, persuasion seems to strengthen the unhappy determination. In one of these cases, the attendants were completely wearied with their endeavours; and on removing the food, one of them took a piece of the meat which had been repeatedly offered to the patient, and threw it under the fire-grate; at the same time, exclaiming, that she should not have it. The poor creature, who seemed governed by the rule of contraries, immediately rushed from her seat, seized the meat from the ashes, and devoured it. For a short time, she was induced to eat, by the attendants availing themselves of this contrary disposition; but it was soon rendered unnecessary, by the removal of this unhappy feature of the disorder.

The attendants at the Retreat, feel themselves in no danger of injury from the patients, who are unconfined; many of whom, previously to their admission, have been accustomed to much severity. No instance has occurred of any serious injury being done by a patient, to any of the attendants; and at no period has there been manifested a general spirit of dissatisfaction, or a tendency to revolt.

The common attendants are not allowed to apply any extraordinary coercion to the patients, by way of punishment, or to change, in any degree, the usual mode of treatment, without the permission of the superintendents. This limitation to their power is of the utmost importance, as it obliges them to seek the good opinion of the patient, and to endeavour to govern rather by the influence of esteem than of severity.

When it is deemed necessary to apply the strait-waistcoat, or any other mode of coercion, to a violent patient, such an ample force is employed, as precludes the idea of resistance from entering the patient's mind; and hence, irritation, or additional excitement, is generally, in a great degree, prevented.

Where such force cannot be obtained, and the case is urgent, courage and confidence will generally overcome the violence of the patient; for the opinion appears to be well founded, that maniacs are seldom truly courageous. The superintendent was one day walking in a field adjacent to the house, in company with a patient, who was apt to be vindictive on very slight occasions. An exciting circumstance occurred. The maniac retired a few paces, and seized a large stone, which he immediately held up, as in the act of throwing at his companion. The superintendent, in no degree ruffled, fixed his eye upon the patient, and in a resolute tone of voice, at the same time advancing, commanded him to lay down the stone. As he approached, the hand of the lunatic gradually sunk from its threatening position, and permitted the stone to drop to the ground. He then submitted to be quietly led to his apartment.

I conceive it useless to enter into more minute details of the modes of coercion and restraint, since experience alone can fully teach the best means of exercising them; and the attendant who possesses a good understanding, and has taken a just view of the character of the insane, will soon perceive for himself, the necessary degree, time, and mode of coercion, which those who are placed under his care require. But they who have had an opportunity of observation, and they only, can conceive the difficulty of entirely subduing the vindictive feelings, which the inconsistent, but often half rational, conduct of the patient, frequently excites in the minds of the inferior attendants.

It is therefore an object of the highest importance, to infuse into the minds of these persons, just sentiments, with regard to the poor objects placed under their care; to impress upon them, that " coercion is only to be considered as a protecting and salutary restraint;" and to remind them, that the patient is really under the influence of a disease, which deprives him of responsibility; and frequently leads him into expressions and conduct the most opposite to his character and natural dispositions.

But even this view of the subject is not exempt from danger; if the attendant does not sufficiently consider the degree in which the pa-

tient may be influenced by moral and rational inducements. These contradictory features in
their character, frequently render it exceedingly
difficult to insure the proper treatment of deranged persons. To consider them at the same
time both as brothers, and as mere automata;
to applaud all they do right; and pity, without
censuring, whatever they do wrong, requires
such a habit of philosophical reflection, and
Christian charity, as is certainly difficult to attain.

OF THE MEANS OF PROMOTING THE GENERAL COMFORT OF THE INSANE.

THE comfort of the patients is therefore considered of the highest importance, in a curative
point of view. The study of the superinten ents
to promote it with all the assiduity of parental,
but judicious attention, has been, in numerous
instances, rewarded by an almost filial attachment. In their conversation with the patients,
they adapt themselves to their particular weak-
ness; but, at the same time, endeavour to draw
them insensibly from the sorrow, or the error,
which marks the disease.

The female superintendent, who possesses an
uncommon share of benevolent activity, and who
has the chief management of the female patients,
as well as of the domestic department, occasionally gives a general invitation to the patients,
to a tea-party. All who attend, dress in their
best clothes, and vie with each other in politeness and propriety. The best fare is provided,
and the visiters are treated with all the attention

of strangers. The evening generally passes in
the greatest harmony and enjoyment. It rarely
happens that any unpleasant circumstance occurs; the patients control in a wonderful degree,
their different propensities; and the scene is at
once curious, and affectingly gratifying.

Some of the patients occasionally pay visits to
the friends in the city; and female visiters are
appointed every month by the committee, to pay
visits to those of their own sex; to converse with
them, and to propose to the superintendents, or
the Committee, any improvements which may
occur to them. The visiters sometimes take tea
with the patients, who are much gratified with
the attention of their friends, and mostly behave
with propriety.

It will be necessary here to mention, that the
visits of former intimate friends, have frequently been attended with disadvantage to the patients; except when convalescence had so far
advanced, as to afford a prospect of a speedy return to the bosom of society. It is, however,
very certain, that as soon as reason begins to
return, the conversation of judicious, indifferent
persons, greatly increases the comfort, and is
considered almost essential to the recovery of
many patients. On this account, the convalescents of every class, are frequently introduced
into the society of the rational parts of the family. They are also permitted to sit up till the
usual time for the family to retire to rest, and
are allowed as much liberty as their state of
mind, will admit.

Those who have had the opportunity of observing the restoration of reason, will be aware,
that she does not, in general, at once, resume

her lost empire over the mind. Her approach resembles rather the gradual influx of the tide; she seems to struggle to advance, but again and again is compelled to recede. During this contest, the judicious attendant, may prove the most valuable ally of reason; and render to her the most essential assistance, in the recovery of her lawful throne.

In some cases, however, the cloud which envelopes the mind is suddenly dispersed, and the patient seems to awake at once as out of a dream. In others the progress of recovery is gradual and uniform.

As indolence has a natural tendency to weaken the mind, and to induce ennui and discontent, every kind of rational and innocent employment is encouraged.

The attendant will soon perceive what kind of employment or amusement, is best adapted to the different patients under his care. He will observe that those of the most active and exciting kind, will be best adapted to the melancholy class, where they can be induced to engage in them; and that the more sedentary employments, are generally preferable for the maniacal class. No strict rule, however, can properly be laid down on this subject; and the inclination of the patient may generally be indulged, except the employment he desires obviously tends to foster his disease. The means of writing, are, on this account, sometimes obliged to be withheld from the patient, as it would only produce continual essays on his peculiar notions; and serve to fix his errors more completely in his mind. Such patients are, however, *occasionally* indulged, as it is found to give them temporary satisfaction ; and to make them more easily led into suitable engagements.

There certainly requires considerable care in the selection of books for the use of the insane. The works of imagination are generally, for obvious reasons, to be avoided ; and such as are in any degree connected with the peculiar notions of the patient, are decidedly objectionable. The various branches of the mathematics and natural science, furnish the most useful class of subjects on which to employ the minds of the insane ; and they should, as much, as possible, be induced to pursue one subject steadily. Any branch of knowledge with which the patient has been previously acquainted, may be resumed with greater ease ; and his disposition to pursue it will be encouraged by the competency which he is able to exhibit.

I met with a striking instance, of the advantage of attention to this point, some years ago. It was related to me by a person of great respectability, who was himself the subject of the case. He stated, that a few years before that time, his mind had been greatly depressed without any apparent cause. The most dismal thoughts continually haunted his mind, and he found the greatest difficulty, in confining his attention, for the shortest time, to one subject. He felt entirely indifferent to his business and his family ; and, of course, he neglected them. It was with great difficulty he was induced to take sufficient food to support life. His body became emaciated, and his mind more and more enfeebled.

In this state, as he was one day musing upon
his miserable condition, he perceived, by the
faint glimmerings of remaining reason, the still
worse state to which he must be reduced, if he
continued to indulge his gloomy reflections and
habits. Alarmed with the prospect of the future,
he resolved to exert the power which he still
possessed to control his unhappy dispositions,
and to regain the habit of attention. For this
purpose, he determined, immediately to apply
himself to mathematics, with which he had been
well acquainted in his youth, and also to admit
a more liberal regimen.

The first attempt to go through the easiest
problem, cost him indescribable labour and pain.
But he persisted in the endeavour; the difficulty of fixing his attention gradually lessened; he
overcame his tendency to abstinence: and very
shortly recovered the use of his faculties and his
former temper of mind.

Perhaps few persons, in the situation which I
have described, would have had the courage to
form such resolutions: and still fewer, the for-
titude to perform them. The case, however,
certainly points out what may possibly be done;
and how important it is, in a curative point of
view, to encourage the patient in steady mental
pursuit.

The managers of this Institution, are far from
imagining that they have arrived at a state of
perfection in the moral treatment of insanity. If
they have made any considerable approaches towards it, their progress has only served to convince them how much more may probably be
effected; and to fill them with regret, that so little ingenuity has hitherto been exerted on the

crease the comforts of insane persons. There is no doubt, that if the same exertions were used for this purpose, as are frequently employed to amuse the vain, the frivolous, and the idle, many more gleams of comfort would be shed over the unhappy existence of lunatics; and the proportion of cures would be still materially increased.

OF THE RULES OF THE ESTABLISHMENT, &c

The object of the Retreat, being to furnish a comfortable shelter for insane persons, as well as to promote their recovery, its original rules made no distinction between old and recent cases; and did not, in any degree, limit the time of patients continuance in the house. The only restriction relates to idiots; and this appears to have been generally understood as applying, chiefly, to cases of original absence of intellect.

In these respects, the circumstances of this establishment, differ materially from those of some of our largest public institutions.

It appears, from the statement of the master of St. Luke's Hospital, made before a Committee of the House of Commons, that, in this Institution, "The average number of patients at one time is 300;" and that "the average number of incurable patients, in the house at one time, is 115." All patients are discharged from this Asylum at the end of the first year; and if not then recovered, may be entered on the incurable list, to be admitted when a vacancy offers; but it appears that only a certain number of this class of patients are permitted to be in the house at one time. The rules of this hospital do not admit patients " troubled with epileptic or convulsive fits."

By the following quotation from Haslam, it appears, that the rules of Bethlem Hospital guard against the admission of old cases : " Although patients who have been afflicted with insanity more than a year, are not admissible into the hospital, to continue there for the usual time of trial for cure, viz. a twelvemonth ; yet, at the discretion of the Committee, they may be received into it from Lady-day to Michaelmas ; at which latter period they are removed. In the course of the last twenty years, seventy-eight patients of this description have been received."

There are, however, a number of patients in Bethlem, who have been there many years ; and I therefore conclude, that a certain proportion is permitted, as in St. Luke's, to remain on the incurable establishment. But, as Haslam states, that from the year 1784 to 1794, out of 1664 cases admitted, 1090 were discharged uncured, I presume that the number of patients in this hospital, who have been afflicted with insanity more than a year, is comparatively very small.

A large majority of the cases admitted into the Retreat, have not been recent. In several instances, the disorder had existed from fifteen to twenty years previously to their admission ; and, of course, no reasonable hope could be entertained of the patient's recovery. The total proportion of cures cannot, therefore, be expected to be large. I will not, however, omit to mention, that the number of these must have been fewer, if the rules had limited the time of continuance in the house, as is the case in the two charitable Institutions above mentioned. But, it must also be observed that several patients who have been insane at the expiration of twelve months, have remained in the house from three to six months longer on probation, or *at their own request*, until a suitable situation offered for them.

Others, who have been apparently well at the end of twelve months, have relapsed before they quitted the house ; and I cannot avoid attributing to the premature discharge of insane persons, many of the relapses which occur after they leave the places provided for their care. Several of the symptoms which mark the disorder in its incipient state, also mark an advanced stage of convalescence. In either case, though no absolute act of insanity is committed, the mind is unable to bear that stimulus or exertion, which would even be salutary to it, in a state of perfect sanity.

APPENDIX.

THE Author hopes he shall be justified in presenting the reader with the sentiments of some respectable persons, who have carefully inspected the Retreat. His view in doing so. is to confirm the testimony which he has given in the preceding pages, of the practices of this Institution, and which might be suspected of partiality, if it were not supported by the evidence of disinterested persons, who were qualified to judge on the occasion.

In the year 1798, Dr. Delarive, of Geneva, after having examined a great number of public and private establishments of a similar nature, visited the Retreat. It was then in its infancy; but, the Doctor was so far pleased with the general management, as to write a very favourable description of it, in a letter addressed to the editors of " The British Library." This letter afterwards appeared on the Continent in a separate form, from a copy of which the following extracts are made.

After describing the evils which have existed in the treatment of the insane in public hospitals, which he observes would lead one to suppose, that madmen were employed in tormenting other madmen, he says, " The respectable society of Quakers have at length endeavoured to remedy these evils ; it has been desirous of securing to those of its members, who should have the unhappiness to lose their reason, without possessing a fortune adequate to have recourse to expensive establishments, all the resources of art, and all the comforts of life, compatible with their situation. A voluntary subscription furnished the funds ; and, about two years since, an establishment, which appears to unite many advantages, with all possible economy, was founded near the city of York.

" If the mind shrinks for a moment at the aspect of this terrible disease, which seems calculated to humble the

G

reason of man; it must afterwards feel pleasing emotions, in considering all that an ingenious benevolence has been able to invent, to cure and comfort the patients afflicted with this malady.

"This house is situated a mile from York, in the midst of a fertile and cheerful country; it presents not the idea of a prison, but rather that of a large rural farm. It is surrounded by a garden. There is no bar or grating to the windows, their place is supplied by a means of which I shall afterwards give an account."

After a general view of the economy of the Retreat, and the general treatment of the patients, the Doctor thus concludes his letter: " You will perceive, that in the moral treatment of the insane, they do not consider them as absolutely deprived of reason; or, in other words, as inaccessible to the motives of fear, hope, feeling and honour. It appears that they consider them rather as children, who have too much strength, and who make a generous use of it. Their punishments and rewards must be immediate, since that which is distant has no effect upon them. A new system of education must be adopted to give a fresh course to their ideas. Subject them at first; encourage them afterwards, employ them, and render their employment agreeable by attractive means. I think that if we could find still stronger means to excite feelings of benevolence in their minds, we should accelerate their recovery by the agreeable emotions which accompany all the affections. But it is evident, that every needless restraint excites in them the vindictive passions, to which they are but too prone, and prolongs the continuance of the disease."

A few years since, W. STARKE, Esq. architect, of Glasgow, who was engaged to prepare a plan of an Asylum for that city and the West of Scotland, visited the Retreat. The following extract is made from his valuable " Remarks on the Construction and Management of Lunatic Asylums," published in the year 1810. " In some Asylums, which I have visited, chains are fixed to every table, and to every bedpost; in others, they are not to be found within the walls. The idea of inflicting corporal punishment is held in abhorrence; and rods or whips are considered as engines of power, too dreadful to be committed to the hands of servants, who may soon convert them into instruments of oppression.

In such asylums, however, there are no appearances of insubordination. The whole demeanour of the patients, on the contrary, is most remarkably submissive and orderly. The one to which I especially allude, the Retreat, or Quaker Asylum, near York, it may be proper to mention, is occupied by a description of people, whose usual habits in life are highly regular and exemplary; but the chief cause of its superiority will be found to lie in the government of the Asylum. It is a government of humanity and of consummate skill, and requires no aid from the arm of violence, or the exertion of brutal force.

At the Retreat, they sometimes have patients brought to them, frantic, and in irons, whom they at once release, and, by mild arguments and gentle arts, reduce almost immediately to obedience and orderly behaviour. A great deal of delicacy appears in the attentions paid to the smaller feelings of the patients. The iron bars, which guarded the windows, have been avoided, and neat iron sashes, having all the appearance of wooden ones, have been substituted in their place; and, when I visited them, the managers were occupied in contriving how to get rid of the bolts with which the patients are shut up at night, on account of their harsh ungrateful sound, and of their communicating to the Asylum somewhat of the air and character of a prison.

The effects of such attentions, both on the happiness of the patients, and the discipline of the Institution, are more important than may at first view be imagined. Attachment to the place and to the managers, and an air of comfort and of contentment, rarely exhibited within the precincts of such establishments, are consequences easily discovered in the general demeanour of the patients.

THE following testimony is extracted from an account lately published of the Lunatic Asylum at Edinburgh; and we are authorised to state, that it comes from the pen of Dr. DUNCAN, senr. who visited the Retreat in the year 1812, after having seen most of the Institutions of a similar nature in Britain.

That the government of the insane requires a certain degree of restraint, both for the safety of the individual and of others, no one can doubt. But very different opinions have been entertained with regard to the utmost degree of coercion, which is necessary in any case. Now, however, this point may be considered as in some degree settled by experience. The fraternity denominated Quakers have demonstrated, beyond contradiction, the very great advantage resulting from a mode of treatment in cases of insanity, much more mild than was before introduced into almost any Lunatic Asylum, either at home or abroad. That fraternity, who have been long and justly celebrated for charity and humanity, have established in the neighbourhood of the city of York, *The Retreat*, as they term it, a building appropriated to deranged members of their own community. In the management of this Institution, they have set an example which claims the imitation, and deserves the thanks, of every sect and every nation. For, without much hazard of contradiction from those acquainted with the subject, it may be asserted, that the Retreat at York, is at this moment the best regulated establishment in Europe, either for the recovery of the insane, or for their comfort, when they are in an incurable state.

Dr. NAUDI, president of the Maltese Hospital, after carefully inspecting the Retreat in the present year, gave the following testimony respecting it:

"I am very glad to have been at York, to observe the Retreat there kept by the Society of Friends. This house, or Retreat, for the trouble in mind, I think is one of the best things I saw in England on the same subject; and having observed many others on the Continent, I dare say that it is the best in all the world. The situation of the building out of the town, a large garden around it, the propriety of the rooms, the cleanliness of the patients, the way which they are kept, as for dressing, as for feeding them, is very remarkable to be observed."*

---

* Dr. N. had studied the English language, only nine months.

THE END.

HINTS

FOR INTRODUCING AN IMPROVED MODE

OF TREATING

THE INSANE

IN THE ASYLUM;

Read before the Governors of the New-York Hospital, on the 4th of Fourth-month, 1815.

—◦✦◦—

BY THOMAS EDDY,

One of the Asylum Committee.

—◦✦◦—

PRINTED FOR THE USE OF THE GOVERNORS.

—◦✦◦—

1815.

HINTS

FOR INTRODUCING

AN

IMPROVED MODE OF TREATING

THE INSANE

IN THE ASYLUM.

—◦✦◦—

OF the numerous topics of discussion, on subjects relating to the cause of humanity, there is none which has stronger claims to our attention, than that which relates to the treatment of the insane.

Though we may reasonably presume, this subject was by no means overlooked by the ancients, we may fairly conclude, it is deservedly the boast of modern times, to have treated it with any degree of success.

It would have been an undertaking singularly interesting and instructive, to trace the different methods of cure which have been pursued in different ages, in the treat-

1 *

ment of those labouring under mental derangement ; and to mark the various results with which they were attended. The
radical defect, in all the different modes of
cure that have been pursued, appears to be,
that of considering mania a *physical* or
bodily disease, and adopting for its removal merely physical remedies. Very lately, however, a spirit of inquiry has been
excited, which has given birth to a new
system of treatment of the insane ; and
former modes of medical discipline, have
now given place to that which is generally denominated *moral management.*

This interesting subject has closely engaged my attention for some years, and I
conceive that the further investigation
of it, may prove highly beneficial to the
cause of humanity, as well as to science, and
excite us to a minute inquiry, how far we
may further contribute to the relief and
comfort of the maniacs placed under our
care. In pursuing this subject, my views
have been much extended, and my mind
considerably enlightened, by perusing the
writings of Doctors Creighton, Arnold,
and Rush ; but, more particularly, the account of the Retreat near York, in England. Under these impressions, I feel
extremely desirous of submitting to the
consideration of the Governors, a plan,
to be adopted by them, for introducing

a system of moral treatment for the lunatics in the Asylum, to a greater extent than has hitherto been in use in this
country. The great utility of confining
ourselves almost exclusively to a course
of moral treatment, is plain and simple,
and incalculably interesting to the cause
of humanity ; and perhaps no work contains so many excellent and appropriate
observations on the subject, as that entitled, *The Account of the Retreat.* The
author, Samuel Tuke, was an active manager of that establishment, and appears to
have detailed, with scrupulous care and
minuteness, the effects of the system pursued towards the patients. I have, therefore, in the course of the following remarks, with a view of illustrating the subject with more clearness, often adopted
the language and opinions of Tuke, but
having frequently mixed my own observation with his, and his manner of expression
not being always adapted to our circumstances and situation, I have attempted to vary the language, so as to
apply it to our own insitution ; this will
account for many of the subsequent remarks not being noticed as taken from
Tuke's work.

It is, in the first place, to be observed, that in most cases of insanity, from

whatever cause it may have arisen, or
to whatever extent it may have proceeded, the patient possesses some
small remains of ratiocination and self-
command ; and although many cannot
be made sensible of the irrationality
of their conduct or opinions, yet they are
generally aware of those particulars, for
which the world considers them proper
objects of confinement. Thus it frequently happens, that a patient, on his first introduction into the asylum, will conceal
all marks of mental aberration ; and, in
some instances, those who before have
been ungovernable, have so far deceived
their new friends, as to make them
doubt their being insane.

It is a generally received opinion, that
the insane who are violent, may be reduced to more calmness and quiet, by exciting the principle of *fear*, and by the use
of chains or corporal punishments. There
cannot be a doubt that the principle of fear
in the human mind, when moderately and
judiciously excited, as it is by the operation of just and equal laws, has a salutary
effect on society. It is of great use in the
education of children, whose imperfect
knowledge and judgment, occasion them
to be less influenced by other motives.
But where fear is *too much* excited, and

especially, when it becomes the chief motive of action, it certainly tends to contract the understanding, weaken the benevolent affections, and to debase the mind. It is, therefore, highly desirable, and more wise, to call into action as much as possible, the operation of superior motives. Fear ought never to be induced, except when an object absolutely necessary cannot be otherwise obtained. Maniacs are often extremely irritable; every care, therefore, should be taken, to avoid that kind of treatment that may have any tendency towards exciting the passions. Persuasion and kind treatment, will most generally supersede the necessity of coercive means. There is considerable analogy between the judicious treatment of children and that of insane persons. Locke has observed, "the great secret of education, is in finding out the way to keep the child's spirit easy, active, and free; and yet, at the same time, to restrain him from many things he has a mind to, and to draw him to things which are uneasy to him." Even with the more violent and vociferous maniacs, it will be found best to approach them with mild and soft persuasion. Every pains should be taken to excite in the patient's mind, a desire of esteem. Though this principle may not be sufficiently powerful to enable them to resist the strong irregular tendency of their disease ; yet, *when properly cultivated*, it may lead many to struggle to overcome and conceal their morbid propensities, or at least, to confine their deviations within such bounds, as do' not make them obnoxious to those about them. This struggle is highly beneficial to the patient ; by strengthening his mind, and conducing to a salutary habit of self-restraint, an object, no doubt, of the greatest importance to the cure of insanity by *moral means.*

It frequently occurs, that one mark of insanity, is a fixed false conception, and a total incapacity of conviction. In *such* cases, it is generally advisable, to avoid reasoning* with them, as it irritates and rivets their false perception more strongly on the mind. On this account, every means ought to be taken to seduce the mind from

---

* The following anecdotes illustrate the observation before made, that maniacs frequently retain the power of reasoning to a certain extent ; and that the discerning physician, may oftentimes successfully avail himself of the remains of this faculty in controling the aberrations of his patient :—A patient, in the Pennsylvania Hospital, who called his physician his father, once lifted his hand to strike him. " What !" said his physician, (Dr. Rush,) with a plaintive tone of voice, " strike your father ?" the madman dropped his arm, and instantly showed marks of contrition for his conduct. The following was related to me by Samuel Coates, president of the Pennsylvania Hospital :—A maniac had made several attempts to set fire to the Hospital : upon being remonstrated with, he said, " I am a sal-

unhappy and favourite musings; and particularly with melancholic patients; they should freely partake of bodily exercises, walking, riding, conversations, innocent sports, and a variety of other amusements; they should be gratified with birds, deer, rabbits, &c. Of all the modes by which maniacs may be induced to restrain themselves, regular employment is perhaps the most efficacious; and those kinds of employment are to be preferred, both on a moral and physical account, which are accompanied by considerable bodily action, most agreeable to the patient, and most opposite to the illusions of his disease.

In short, the patient should be always treated as much like a *rational* being as the state of his mind will possibly allow. In order that he may display his knowledge to the best advantage, such topics should be introduced as will be most likely to interest him; if he is a mechanic or agriculturalist, he should be asked questions relating to his art, and consulted, upon any occasion in which his knowledge may be useful. These considerations are

amander;" "but recollect," said my friend Coates, "all the patients in the house are not salamanders;" "That is true," said the maniac, and never afterwards attempted to set fire to the Hospital.

Many similar instances of a degree of reason being retained by maniacs, and some of cures effected by pertinent and well directed conversations, are to be met with in the records of medical writers.

undoubtedly very material, as they regard the comforts of insane persons ; but they are of far greater importance as they relate to the cure of the disorder. The patient, feeling himself of some consequence, is induced to support it by the exertion of his reason, and by restraining those dispositions, which if indulged, would lesson the respectful treatment he wishes to receive, or lower his character in the eyes of his companions and attendants.

Even when it is absolutely necessary to employ coercion, if on its removal the patient promises to control himself, great reliance may frequently be placed upon his word, and under this engagement, he will be apt to hold a successful struggle with the violent propensities of his disorder. Great advantages may also be derived, in the moral management of maniacs, from an acquaintance with the previous employment, habits, manners, and prejudices of the individual : this may truly be considered as indispensably necessary to be known, as far as can be obtained ; and, as it may apply to each case, should be registered in a book, for the inspection of the Committee of the Asylum, and the physician ; the requisite information should be procured immediately on the admission of each patient; the mode of procuring it will be spoken of hereafter.

Nor must we forget to call to our aid, in endeavouring to promote self-restraint, the mild but powerful influence of the precepts of our holy religion. Where these have been strongly imbued in early life, they become little less than principles of our nature ; and their restraining power is frequently felt, even under the delirious excitement of insanity. To encourage the influence of religious principles over the mind of the insane, may be considered of great consequence, as a means of cure, provided it be done *with great care and circumspection*. For this purpose, as well as for reasons still more important, it would certainly be right, to promote in the patient, *as far as circumstances would permit*, an attention to his accustomed modes of paying homage to his Maker.

In pursuing the desirable objects above enumerated, we ought not to expect too suddenly to reap the good effects of our endeavours; nor should we too readily be disheartened by occasional disappointments. It is necessary to call into action, as much as possible, every remaining power and principle of the mind, and to remember, that, " in the wreck of the intellect, the affections very frequently survive." Hence, the necessity of considering *the degree* in which the patient may be influenced by moral and rational inducements.

The contradictory features in their characters, frequently render it exceedingly difficult to insure the proper treatment of insane persons; to pursue this with any hopes of succeeding, so that we may in any degree ameliorate their distressed condition, renders it indispensably necessary that attendants only should be chosen who are possessed of good sense, and of amiable dispositions, clothed as much as possible with philosophical reflection, and above all, with that love and charity that mark the humble christian.

Agreeably to these principles, I beg leave to suggest the following regulations to be adopted, in accomplishing the objects in view :

1st. No patient shall hereafter be confined by chains.

2nd. In the most violent states of mania, the patient should be confined in a room with the windows, &c. closed, so as nearly to exclude the light, and kept confined, if necessary, in a strait jacket, so as to walk about the room or lie down on the bed at pleasure ; or by straps, &c. he may,

particularly if there appears in the patient
a strong determination to self-destruction,
be confined on the bed, and the apparatus
so fixed as to allow him to turn and otherwise change his position.

3d. The power of judicious kindness to
be generally exercised, may often be blessed with good effects, and it is not till after
other moral remedies are exercised, that
recourse should be had to restraint, or the
power of fear on the mind of the patient;
yet it may be proper sometimes, by way
of punishment, to use the shower bath.

4th. The common attendants shall not
apply any extraordinary coercion by way
of punishment, or change in any degree
the mode of treatment prescribed by
the physician; on the contrary, it is
considered as their indispensable duty, to
seek by acts of kindness the good opinion
of the patients, so as to govern them by
the influence of esteem rather than of severity.

5th. On the first day of the week, the
superintendant, or the principal keeper of
the Asylum, shall collect as many of the
patients as may appear to them suitable,
and read some chapters in the Bible.

6th. When it is deemed necessary to
apply the strait-jacket, or any other mode
of coercion, by way of punishment or

restraint, such an ample force should be employed as will preclude the idea of resistance from entering the mind of the patient.

7th. It shall be the duty of the deputy keeper, immediately on a patient being admitted, to obtain his name, age, where born, what has been his employment or occupation, his general disposition and habits, when first attacked with mania; if it has been violent or otherwise, the cause of his disease, if occasioned by religious melancholy, or a fondness for ardent spirits, if owing to an injury received on any part of the body, or supposed to arise from any other known cause, hereditary or adventitious, and the name of the physician who may have attended him, and his manner of treating the patient while under his direction.

8th. Such of the patients as may be selected by the physician, or the committee of the Asylum, shall be occasionally taken out to walk or ride under the care of the deputy keeper : and it shall be also his duty to employ the patients in such manner, and to provide them with such kinds of amusements and books as may be approved and directed by the Committee.

9th. The female keeper shall endeavour to have the female patients constantly em-

ployed at suitable work ; to provide proper amusements, books, &c. to take them
out to walk as may be directed by the
Committee.

10th. It shall be the indispensable duty
of the keepers, to have all the patients as
clean as possible in their persons, and to
preserve great order and decorum when
they sit down to their respective meals.

11th. It shall be the duty of the physician to keep a book, in which shall be entered an historical account of each patient,
stating his situation, and the medical and
moral treatment used ; which book shall
be laid before the Committee, at their
weekly meetings.

The sentiments and improvements proposed in the preceding remarks, for the
consideration of the governors, are adapted to our present situation and circumstances ; but a further and more extensive
improvement has occurred to my mind,
which I conceive, would very considerably conduce towards effecting the cure,
and materially ameliorate the condition
and add to the comfort of the insane ; at
the same time that it would afford an ample opportunity of ascertaining how far
that disease may be removed by moral
management alone, which it is believed,

will, in many instances, be more effectual in
controling the maniac, than medical treatment, especially, in those cases where the
disease has proceeded from causes operating directly on the mind.

I would propose, that a lot, not less than
ten acres, should be purchased by the
governors, conveniently situated, within a
few miles of the city, and to erect a sub-
stantial building, on a plan calculated for
the accommodation of fifty lunatic patients; the ground to be improved in such
a manner as to serve for agreeable walks,
gardens, &c. for the exercise and amusement of the patients : this establishment
might be placed under the care and superintendance of the Asylum Committee, and
be visited by them once every week : a
particular description of patients to remain at this Rural Retreat ; and such
others, who might appear as suitable objects, might be occasionally removed there
from the Asylum.

The cost, and annual expense of sup-
porting this establishment, is a matter of
small consideration, when we duly consider the important advantages it would
afford to a portion of our fellow-creatures,
who have such strong claims on our sympathy and commiseration.

But, it is a fact that can be satisfactorily demonstrated, that such an establishment would not increase our expenses; and, moreover, would repay us even the interest of the money that might be necessary to be advanced, for the purchase of the ground and erecting the buildings. The board of the patients (supposing fifty) would yield two hundred dollars per week, or ten thousand four hundred dollars per annum.

Supposing the ground, building, &c. to cost $50,000, the interest on this sum, at 6 per cent. would be $3000, there would yet remain $7400, for the maintenance and support of the establishment; a sum larger than would be required for that purpose.

We had lately in the Asylum, more than ninety patients; and, at that time, had repeated applications to receive an additional number; the Committee, however, concluded, that as the building was not calculated to accommodate more than seventy-five, it would be an act of injustice to take in any more; they, therefore, concluded to reduce the number to seventy-five, and strictly to refuse receiving any beyond that number. This may serve clearly to show, that we might safely calculate, that we should readily have applications to accommodate one hundred and twenty-five patients.

This succinct view of the subject may suffice, at this time, as outlines of my plan; and which is respectfully submitted to the governors, for their consideration.

PROPOSALS

FOR ESTABLISHING A

RETREAT FOR THE INSANE,

TO BE CONDUCTED BY

GEORGE PARKMAN, M. D.

———

"Ces asiles des malheurs des mortels
Sont du Bon Dieu les meilleurs autels."

———

BOSTON :

PRINTED BY JOHN ELIOT, NO. 5, COURT STREET

———

1814.

A RETREAT FOR INSANE PERSONS

Is to be established on one of the most delightful and retired spots, near Boston.

Application for admission into it may be made immediately to Dr. Parkman.

No time will be lost in making preparations for the accommodation of each applicant, as his or her circumstances may require.

Accommodations will be made for those patients, for whom the occasional or constant residence of a friend or attendant with them is adviseable.

Expenses will be proportioned to each patient's pecuniary situation, and to his demands on the Institution. The expenses will not exceed those in similar establishments.

The object of the Institution has been a subject of the particular attention of the Physician from the commencement of his professional pursuits. He has visited most of the establishments for the Insane of Our Country, of the British empire, of France, Italy and Switzerland; and he has formed such connexion with them, as will give him early information of improvements, which shall be adopted in them.

It is proposed to call the Establishment "the Retreat;" or by some name, which will not excite any unpleasant ideas.

It is hoped, that the mention of it will recall to the minds of those, who shall have resided in it, a place, where they have found a friend, indefatigable in his exertions to render them happy, and to restore them to usefulness.

To those, who may be candidates for residence in the Retreat, it is hoped, that it may be considered a delightful temporary abode, affording superiour advantages for establishing health, or for diversion and respite from perplexing cares.

The arrangement of the house will resemble, as much as possible, that of a private residence, affording as many enjoyments of social life, as the circumstances of each patient may allow; so that the idea of a hospital, or of any thing like it, may not intrude itself.

The patient will be courteously received at the Retreat, as a stranger, and he shall not discover that his misfortune is known there, until maniacal extravagance demands his restraint.

The Physician will be assiduous in acquiring early knowledge of his patient, to meet with judgment the first sally of his disorder.

Every thing, relating to the Establishment, will be particularly directed by the Physician. No person will be employed in it, who is not completely dependant on him, and none shall have an opportunity of repeating a breach of duty.

The proposed Institution has not the means of extending its influence to objects of charity. It will be ever ready to second the views of the charitable. Should any sums be appropriated by individuals, or by publick bodies, for the Insane Poor, this Institution will receive them, under such conditions, as may answer the ends of the Donors.

General experience, in the treatment of insanity, has furnished the following results, which will be kept constantly in view, in the management of this Institution.

'Maniacs are under the influence of a disease which deprives them of responsibility; and frequently leads them to conduct, opposite to their character and dispositions. Their extravagances should be considered but as the impulses of an automaton, no more calculated to excite anger, than is a blow from a stone propelled by its gravity. To punish the misconduct, however extravagant, of a man, who avows his inability to govern his actions, would be cruel. Attempts to rectify errours, the absurdity of which he is ready to acknowledge and lament, would be of but little advantage.

That it is necessary to commence acquaintance with lunatics, by exhibition of strength, or appearance of austerity; that madness, in all its forms, is

capable of entire control, by excitement of fear, is
an errour, strengthened by indifference to the comforts of the Insane, and by having rendered coercion
necessary by unkind treatment.

To detain maniacs in constant seclusion, and to
load them with chains ; to leave them defenceless,
to the brutality of underlings, on pretence of danger, from their extravagances ; to rule them with a
rod of iron, as if to shorten their existence, already
wretched ; is a superintendence, more distinguished for its convenience, than for its humanity or its
success. If " oppression makes a wise man mad,"
will stripes and injuries, for which the receiver
knows no cause, make a mad man wise ; or will they
exasperate his disease and excite his resentment ?

There are patients, who may be made to obey
their attendants, with promptitude—to rise, to sit, to
stand, to walk, or run at their pleasure, though expressed by a look only. Such obedience, and
even the appearance of affection, we see in the
poor animals, who are exhibited to gratify curiosity in natural history. But who can avoid reflecting, in observing such spectacles, that the readiness,
with which the tiger obeys his master, is from treatment, at which humanity shudders ?

That the continual or frequent excitement of
fear should " bid melancholy cease to mourn," is
an idea too absurd to require the refutation of practice. But there has been too much experience on

this subject; hence we may, in a great degree, explain, why melancholy has been considered so much less susceptible of care than mania. But where mild treatment has been adopted, a large portion of melancholy patients has recovered.

Maniacs, who have been brought to the Asylum, represented uncommonly furious, rendered so probably, by severity, have, on being received with affability, soothed by consolation and sympathy, and encouraged to expect a happier lot, subsided into a placid coolness, to which has succeeded rapid convalescence.

Those, who pursue the terrific system of management, should reflect on the awful responsibility attached to their conduct. But those only, who have had opportunities of observing, can conceive the difficulty of entirely subduing the vindictive feelings, which the inconsistent, but sometimes half-rational conduct of the patient often excites in the minds of ordinary attendants. To consider the insane, at the same time as brothers, and as mere automata; to applaud all they do right; and to pity, without censuring, whatever they do wrong, requires a habit of reflection, difficult to attain.

This Institution will aim to avoid every thing, which can excite or aggravate the fury or sadness of the patients; to appear not to notice their extravagances; to yield to their caprices, with apparent complacency; to elude with dexterity their inconsiderate demands; to draw them insensibly from the sorrow, or the errour, which marks their disease : to give them impulses, with such address as to impress them with the conviction that they originate with themselves ; to soothe them by kind treatment, consolatory language, and particularly by encouraging hope ; and to render all these means effective by dispassionate firmness. Coercion exerted towards the patients shall appear to be only a protecting and salutary restraint, the result of necessity, reluctantly resorted to, and commensurate with the violence or petulance it is intended to correct, avoiding, as far as possible, whatever irritates or degrades the feelings.

Such coercion seldom exasperates violence, or produces that feverish and sometimes furious irritability, in which the maniacal character is completely developed, and under which all power of self-control is lost. But, where fear is too much excited. and where it becomes the chief motive of action, it tends to contract the understanding, and to weaken the benevolent affections. It is determined, in this Establishment, to excite, as much as possible, the operation of superiour motives ; and fear shall not be induced, but when a necessary object cannot otherwise be obtained.

The Institution will possess force calculated to master the extravagances of the patients, and to preclude the idea of resistance.

9

Insane persons generally possess a degree of control over their wayward propensities. This is often exercised before strangers. The patient is induced to support his consequence, by restraining those propensities, which, if indulged, would lessen the respect, he receives. Attention to this circumstance may be rendered exceedingly important, during the first part of a patient's residence in the Institution. The Physician will assiduously encourage every effort to self-restraint in his patients, so that habit may strengthen their power of controlling their disorder.

An important part of management with those who have been most happy in the treatment of Insanity, has consisted in giving full employment to the remaining faculties of the lunatic, and in engaging them about objects, opposite to their illusions.

The lost faculties often recover themselves, when an object is presented, calculated to fix the attention.

Indolence weakens the mind, and induces *ennui* and discontent. Salutary exercises and employments render the labourers cheerful, and fit them for repose at night.

In this institution, employments will be encouraged, by the prospect of recompense, or by other motives. The establishment will possess extensive enclosures, where those, whose circumstances will admit, may be engaged in gardening, &c.

The first ray of returning reason will be seized with avidity, and tenderly fostered.

Those apartments, in the establishment, which command open and cheerful scenery, will be allotted to melancholics, in preference to any other patients.

Attention will be given to prevent the contagious influence of acts of maniacal extravagance. Confirmed mania will never be exposed to the sight of patients, recently and perhaps transiently deranged. Ideotism will never be exposed to the other classes of patients : nor will any of the insane be exposed to the unfeeling curiosity of visitors.

In New England, but little ingenuity has been exerted to increase the comforts of the Insane, or to procure his recovery. He has, in many instances, been left to subsist on bread and water, and to lie on straw, chained in a dark, solitary and loathsome cell, experiencing no solicitude in his fate, and a victim of an idle and sometimes interested maxim, that "insanity is incurable." His personal liberty has been taken from him, perhaps by his nearest relative or dearest friend, whose occasional reproaches have wounded him deeply. The idea of being under restraint, in a place, where he perhaps considers himself master, is constantly irritating him ; and his distress is aggravated, by the brutality of his attendants. Rendered susceptible of the liveliest emotions, by morbid excitement of his nervous system, he gives himself up to all the extravagances of manaical fury, or sinks into the lowest depths of despondence and melancholy.

Many instances, in which the malevolent dispositions are apparent, may be traced to secondary causes, arising from the peculiar circumstances of the patient, or from the management.

A patient, confined at home, naturally feels resentment, when those, whom he has been accustomed to command, refuse to obey, or attempt to restrain him. We may attribute, in part, to similar causes, the indifference to the accustomed sources of dometick pleasure, the disgust towards the tenderest connexions, which are frequently early symptoms of insanity. The maniac is frequently unconscious of his disease. He is unable to account for the change in the conduct of his friends. They appear to him cruel, disobedient, and ungrateful. His disease aggravates their conduct in his view, and leads him to unfounded suspicions. Hence, the estrangement of his affections may frequently be the consequence of either the proper and necessary, or of the mistaken conduct of his friends towards him. Yet, the existence of the benevolent affections, in such cases, is often evidenced, by the patient's attachment to those, who have the immediate care of him, and who treat him with judgment and humanity. Even in those instances where the ingenious humanity of the Superintendent fails to conciliate, and the discase changes the aspect of nature, and represents all mankind as the leagued enemies of the patient, the existence of the social affections is often evidenced, by his attachment to some inferiour animals.

In most cases of insanity, originating in deviation from virtue, the degree of morbid effect, on the intellect, is proportioned to the consciousness of shame, and to the remaining virtue of the victim.

It has been said, by one, who has been a long time conversant with the Insane, I have nowhere seen fonder husbands, more affectionate parents, more pure and exalted patriots, than in the Lunatic Asylum, during their intervals of calmness and reason. A man of sensibility may daily witness there scenes of indescribable tenderness, and of most estimable virtue.

The Superintendent of an Asylum for the Insane should possess mildness, and firmness of manners, the vigilance of an affectionate friend, knowledge of the mind, zeal and sagacity in the discharge of the duties of his office.'

These high qualifications will be the constant aim of the Superintendent of the Proposed Institution. He is encouraged by the support and advice of his Professional Fathers.

The Trustees of the Mass. General Hospital have individually expressed Their warmest approbation of this plan of establishing a Retreat for the Insane, and Their best wishes for its success.

A

DISCOURSE

ON

MENTAL PHILOSOPHY

AS CONNECTED WITH

MENTAL DISEASE,

DELIVERED BEFORE THE

Massachusetts Medical Society,

JUNE 2, 1830

———

BY RUFUS WYMAN, M. D.

Fellow of the Society.

BOSTON:

FROM THE OFFICE OF THE DAILY ADVERTISER.

———————

1830.

MENTAL PHILOSOPHY

AS CONNECTED WITH

MENTAL DISEASE.

Fellows of the
Massachusetts Medical Society ;

You had expected, at your last meeting, an address
from Dr John Gorham. From him you had hoped
to receive instruction and delight. This expectation,
and this hope were disappointed by his death. He
was suddenly cut down in the vigor of manhood and
season of usefulness. Another departed slowly, full of
days, and covered with honors, and learning, and
virtues of the steady growth of a hundred years. Other
fellows, within the same year, went down to the
grave in unusual numbers. And again during the last
year, they were followed by others to be counted with
the dead.

Of the dead, many were your active and useful officers. They were cultivators of sound learning, promoters of the public good, guardians of the public
health, ornaments of human nature. Of these time
will not permit me even to repeat the names. But
the name of Gorham is too intimately connected with
the services of this day, too much honored by the fellows of this society, too much known by the lovers of
medical science, and too dear to the friends of virtue,
not to be mentioned, on this occasion, with the greatest respect. I am not to attempt his eulogy. It was

pronounced over his mortal remains, by his learned and distinguished friend. It issued from the pulpit, and the press. It came spontaneously, and universally from the hearts of the people of this extended city. He was learned, and wise, and good. He was, therefore, valued and loved while living; honored and respected when dead.

The nature of the change, produced in man by death, has ever been a subject of anxious inquiry. The funeral ceremonies of the ancients clearly indicate a belief in them, that their deceased friends continued to exist beyond the grave. Unless the dead had been supposed to have knowledge of the actions of the living, these ceremonies would have been a senseless show.* Whether this belief were derived from early revelation, transmitted by tradition, or from an induction from facts without us, or from a peculiar consciousness or feeling within us, it has existed among the learned, and deep thinkers of almost every age. It has generally been believed, that the substance, to which consciousness, knowledge, and feeling belong, is totally distinct from the body, which we commit to the earth, there to be decomposed and to enter into new combinations, according to chemical laws. But the determination of the question, whether consciousness, thinking, and feeling be attributes of matter or of spirit, seems not to be important in determining the question of man's future existence; for whatever substance it may be, which has existence, knowledge, and feeling here, the same may exist, and know, and feel hereafter.

* Cicero.

The brain is admitted to be an organ, by whose agency we have connexion with the external world. By this agency sensations are produced, and volitions are executed. We have no difficulty in believing, that an impression upon an organ of sense may be transmitted to the brain ; because in this case we can trace a continuity of organized matter. But that there should arise in the brain itself, thus affected, any consciousness or knowledge, is a fact so entirely distinct from, and so destitute of analogy to other affections of matter, as to indicate the existence of some other substance, possessing different properties, or susceptibilities. So in the execution of our volitions, there is for a similar reason, no difficulty in believing, that a change or motion, existing in the brain, may be transmitted to the voluntary organs. That the brain should originate voluntary motion, is to me wholly incomprehensible. But a review of the arguments, advanced by the materialists and immaterialists, would be of little interest on this occasion. Avoiding then the discussion of a question, in which so many have been bewildered, it will be sufficient to notice the *phenomena* of nature.

Powers, faculties, operations, functions and states of mind are terms which are frequently used. Nothing more is expressed by them than bare phenomena, made known to each individual by his own consciousness ; and consciousness itself merely expresses a fact, which can be explained only by reference to the experience of its subject.

We learn then by experience, that man is a being that thinks and feels. Each individual being himself conscious, that he is at different times in different states, is so constituted as to infer from this fact, that others have a similar experience in regard to themselves. These different states, such as perceiving, remembering, comparing, and discerning, and also the different states in anger, joy, hatred, &c. constitute the phenomena, which are called *mental.** They are as closely connected with each other in one clearly marked group or assemblage, as the phenomena, which are common to vegetable and animal life, are connected in another. They are as distinct in their character from the organic phenomena of vegetables and animals, as the organic are from the physical. Nor are the organic actions more interesting to the physician, than should be the mental operations. There is a natural and fixed course of each, which is denominated perfect health.—' *Mens sana in corpore sano.*'

There is a difficulty, and perhaps an impossibility of defining disease of mind ; yet the difficulty seems not to be greater, than in disease of body. The state of perfect health is taken as the standard for each. Every deviation from this state is, strictly speaking, a disease. The deviations in the organic functions, however, are not usually considered diseases, unless they should be attended with pain, uneasiness, or other inconvenience. Neither are the deviations in the mental states or operations of one man to be considered as amounting to disease, unless they be obviously inconsistent with the feelings, judgment, or belief of other men, who are competent judges; so that the mutual

* See Note A.

adaptation, by which one mind is fitted to act in concert with others, is destroyed. It may be objected, that there are no mental diseases. That it is an 'unphilosophical notion, which supposes an immaterial principle, the soul, sick or deranged.'* It is admitted, that an immaterial agent cannot have organic disease ; because it is not composed of material organs. But that the operations, functions, or states of such an agent cannot deviate from their established course, and usual order, is contrary to obvious facts, of which, I think, every individual must at times be conscious.

In *science* men may differ—may adopt peculiar, and sometimes very singular opinions ; yet they may not be accounted insane. Long after Sir Isaac Newton had proved, that the earth is flattened at its poles, the author of the Studies of Nature, contended that it is there elongated ; but he was not adjudged to be a lunatic. After him Capt. Symmes believed, that it was neither flattened, nor elongated. He affirmed, that instead of solid earth, there was a vast hole, forming an entrance into an immense cavern, leaving the earth a mere shell, inhabited, as well on its internal, as its external surface ; yet perhaps Capt. Symmes is entitled to a judgment, as favorable as that of St Pierre.

There are mental deviations, however, which relate to the *ordinary* affairs of life and the daily experience of all, in which no man can depart much from the usual opinions, or conduct of mankind without actual derangement. It is true any man may err from want of information, or experience. But a man of sound mind, will be susceptible of the influence of evidence.

* Combe's Phrenol. add. by Editor, p. 412. Spurzheim on Insanity, p. 101.

He will attend to the arguments against his erroneous opinions, and be willing to correct them.

A deranged man will seldom attend to arguments, or feel the force of evidence against his opinions. He will hold fast a belief, which every rational mind would perceive to be founded on error and falsehood. False belief—delusion is, in view of criminal law, essential to insanity. Lord Erskine, in his defence of Hadfield is most full and clear on this subject, and the court unanimously assented to his exposition. James Hadfield was tried in the Court of King's Bench for shooting at the king in Drury-lane theatre. 'He imagined that he had constant intercourse with the Almighty Author of all things—that the world was coming to a conclusion, and that, like our blessed Savior, he was to sacrifice himself for its salvation, and because he would not be guilty of suicide, though called upon by the imperious voice of heaven, he wished that by the appearance of crime, that his life might be taken from him by others.' His delusion consisted in his belief, that he was under a special command of God—in his belief, that the end of the world was at hand, and in his further belief, that his death would procure its salvation.

In this city, a man believed himself to be King Charles II. He wore a long beard, as was the fashion in the days of that prince. He spoke in the royal style, and required of all persons to address him in language suited to the royal presence. He assumed great dignity of manner, and deemed the touching of his beard the greatest insult. These singularities in conduct did not constitute his derangement. They

9

were indeed proofs of it. His belief, that he was a king, was his delusion. His actions were perfectly consistent with his belief. It would have been unreasonable in him to have conducted differently. His belief, founded on error, did as really govern his conduct, as does the belief of other men, founded on truth, govern theirs.

Last winter an intelligent gentleman believed, that various evil minded persons, who were strangers to him, had often attacked him in the streets with chlorine gas, and had contrived to throw it into his chamber; that it produced pains in his head, and soreness of his nose. He made the doors of his house doubly secure with additional bolts, and caulked the windows, and kept pledgets of lint in his nostrils and ears. This man was the only proper judge of the existence of the pains and soreness. They were feelings, of which he alone could be conscious. But in assigning causes of these feelings, others were equally competent judges; yet contrary to the unanimous opinion of numerous friends, in whom he had great confidence, he continued in the same belief, and frequently and secretly changed his lodgings to escape the annoyance. He said to his friends, 'I know that it appears to you unreasonable, and imaginary, but to me it is a reality; to you it is a proof of insanity, to me it is a source of suffering.'

Lawyers may trace insanity to delusion, and proof of delusion may always be necessary in courts of criminal law to establish the existence of actual derangement. But physicians should extend their inquiries further, and endeavor to ascertain the difference between a state of delusion, and a state of sound mind—

2

to ascertain how a state of delusion or false belief is produced. This inquiry is not less important in the investigation of mental diseases, than is the accurate discrimination of the healthy and disordered states of the organic functions in the investigation of their diseases. A knowledge of the mental functions in health can be derived only from the history of mental operations. This history of facts, with the laws and principles deduced therefrom by the aid of a sound logic, is called the *philosophy of mind*.

Mental philosophy, then, is an indispensable study of an accomplished physician. Such are the mutual dependencies and influences of the mental and organic functions, that diseases of either cannot be well treated without a knowledge of both.* But I would not go back to the vagaries of the ancient metaphysicians. It is sufficient to begin with Locke, and proceed with Brown, Stewart, and Reid. If the reading be confined to a single volume, it may be Payne's Elements of Mental and Moral Science. These writers have been guided by the precepts of Bacon. They have taken facts and sought for their connexions and dependencies. They have labored to become simply the interpreters of nature. Whoever will turn his thoughts within him, and attend to the operations or different states of his own mind, will find in their works a record of mental phenomena, of which his own experience will afford the fullest confirmation. An acquaintance with their writings will fix the philosophical import of many terms in popular and scientific use, concerning which there is much confusion and ambi-

* See Note B.

guity in medical books. The *faculties* of the mind, for example, are usually considered as distinct agents. This is erroneous. The faculties are not parts of the mind. The mind cannot be divided. There is but one agent acting in different ways, or performing different acts. This is the doctrine of the immortal Essay Concerning Human Understanding.* The same doctrine is taught by various authors. Mr Locke, speaking of the understanding and will, says the word faculties must not be ' supposed, (as I suspect it has been,) to stand for some real beings in the soul, that performed those actions of understanding and volition. For when we say the will is the commanding and superior faculty of the soul, that it is or is not free, that it determines the inferior faculties, that it follows the dictates of the understanding, &c. though these and the like expressions, by those who carefully attend to their own ideas, and conduct their thoughts more by the evidence of things, than by the sound of words, may be understood in a clear and distinct sense ; yet I suspect, I say, that this way of speaking of the faculties has misled many into a confused notion of so many distinct agents in us which had their several provinces and authorities, and did command, obey, and perform several actions as so many distinct beings. Which has been no small occasion of wrangling, obscurity, and uncertainty in questions relating to them.'

The very learned Dr Good† says of the faculties, 'we sometimes, however, are apt to speak of them as distinct and separate existences from the mind, or as

* B. 2, ch. 21, § 6.
† Study of Medicine, Cooper's edition, Vol. IV. p. 45.

possessing a sort of independent entity, and as controlling one another by their individual authorities.' Again, 'The faculties of the mind are so many powers.' 'But the power to do one action is not operated upon by the power to do another action.' Yet he says, under the genus Ecphronia, and not very consistently, 'a sound mind supposes an existence of all the mind's feelings and intellectual powers in a state of vigor, and under the *subordination* of the judgment, which is designed by nature to be the *governing or controlling* principle.'*

That the study of mental philosophy is a necessary part of a medical education, will be more apparent by attending to the description of insanity by any approved author. Diseases, affecting the intellect, are placed by Dr Good in his fourth class, under the first order, Phrenica, in which they are thus described ; 'Error, perversion, or debility of one or more of the mental faculties.' The import of these terms must be understood, or the description will be of no use. From this description we learn first, that there are several mental faculties. Then arises the inquiry, what is their number, and what is the character of each ? We next learn, that there may be error, or perversion of one or more of these faculties. Then comes another inquiry, what is their sound state ? for unless this can be ascertained, it will be impossible to know when there is error or perversion. When we have acquired accurate knowledge of the sound state, we can, by comparing the two states, learn in what

* Idem. p. 51.

respects the diseased states deviate from a state of health.

The same learned author proceeds in his description, and remarks, under the genus Ecphronia, or insanity, that there is 'diseased perception with little derangement of the judgment,' &c. The medical student would certainly inquire, what are the mental functions or states, intended by perception and judgment. Unless he do this, he cannot understand the description. Dugald Stewart* observes, that 'in ordinary language we apply the same word, *perception*, to the knowledge, which we have by our senses, of external objects, and to our knowledge of speculative truth; and yet an author would be justly censured who should treat of these two operations of the mind under the same article of perception.' In the definite and philosophical use of the term, perception denotes that mental function, which refers to an external object as its cause, the impression made upon an organ of sensation. Thus when we have a certain impression upon the ear, followed by a sensation, we refer it to a man cutting wood with an axe. But there is another use of the same term, perception,† when we speak of the perception of the agreement or disagreement of two ideas, or of the perception of the relation of the successive steps of a geometrical demonstration, &c. Dr Good has adopted both uses of this word in the proem to his fourth class.‡ In his description of the genus Ecphronia of the same class,

* Elements, Vol. I. ch. 3.

† Consciousness, or discernment, is the proper term.

‡ See also Dr Good's Lucret. De Rerum Natura, Vol. II. p. 110.

I think, it is nowhere pointed out in which of these senses, or in what sense it is to be understood.

Writers on mental philosophy arrange the mental operations or states under two heads, one of which regards our knowledge, the other our feelings. The former includes the functions of intellect, or the intellectual powers or states. The latter includes the affections, emotions or passions, or the pathetical powers or states. Pope, in his Essay on Man, has very happily pointed out this distinction.

> "Two principles in human nature reign,
> Self-love [passion] to urge, and reason to restrain."
> "Man but for that no action could attend,
> And but for this were active to no end."
> "On life's vast ocean diversely we sail,
> Reason the card, but passion is the gale."
> "Love, hope and joy, fair pleasure's smiling train;
> Hate, fear and grief, the family of pain.
> These, mixt with art, and to due bounds confined,
> Make and maintain the balance of the mind."

This division of the mental states or functions has suggested a corresponding division of mental diseases—diseases of the intellect and diseases of the passions.* The same division is the basis of Dr Good's arrangement of the mental disorders, which is clear and comprehensive, and should be thoroughly studied. He has, however, made many subdivisions, more important, perhaps, to a systematic work, than to the treatment of mental diseases.

In diseases of the intellectual functions there may

---

* The term *passion* is here used in an extended sense, including *emotions* and *affections* of various authors.

be perversion, diminution, or augmentation of one or more of the intellectual states or faculties.

1. It has already been observed, that *delusion* or *false belief* exists in all cases of insanity, in the legal meaning of the term. True belief is founded on some intuitive knowledge, some original principles, some self-evident truths, from which, by the process of reasoning, conclusions are derived, to which assent is given. Thus my belief, that the sun will rise again, is an inference from a confidence in the *permanency* of the order of nature. My belief of the existence of an external world is derived from my *sensations*. My belief, that Dr Holyoke lived in Salem, A. D. 1828, arises from my confidence in the evidence of *memory*. My belief, that he was then one hundred years old, arose from my confidence in *testimony*.

If there be perversion in the original principles of belief, all consequential belief will be false. If these foundations of intellect be overturned, the superstructure will be in ruins. The physician and patient cannot meet on common ground. Reasoning will be vain. They are at variance about first principles, which *are not susceptible of proof*, and *do not admit of argument*. Insane persons usually reason right ; but the conclusions are wrong, because the premises are false.

There may be perversion not only in regard to fundamental principles of belief, but there may also be error, in a degree amounting to disease in the faculties exercised in reasoning from these principles. Inferences, which every sound mind would discover to be false, are sometimes made by lunatics from premises, which are true.

2. That there is often a *diminution* of intellectual power, in a degree amounting to disease, comes within the experience of some, and the observation of all. The memory may be imperfect, the agreement or disagreement between ideas may not be discerned, or the mental operations may be slow and unequal.

3. An *augmentation* of one or more of the intellectual powers is another deviation from a state of sound mind. That it is a disease, may perhaps be denied ; and if it be a disease, many might wish to be sick. The disease consists, not in a proportional and permanent augmentation of each faculty, but in the temporary excess of vigor and activity of one or more of the faculties above their just proportion. In some, the quickness and extent of the memory is increased ; in some, the imagination is too active ; in some, there is increased talent of ridicule and sarcasm ; in some, there is a hurry and quickness in all the intellectual operations.

The augmentation of intellectual power is sometimes sudden and wonderful. A gentleman of moderate mental endowments, who played an indifferent game at chess, became deranged in 1819. There was at first some doubt as to the reality of his insanity. On a certain evening he came from his room with a blanket over his shoulders, in the character of an Indian chief ; his head elevated, his body very erect, his step long and firm. His whole manner had an air of dignity, and conscious superiority. He took his seat at a table, upon which was a chess-

board, and played several games with several persons,
by whom he had often, if not usually, been beaten.
But he was now conqueror in almost every game. He
played with a skill and quickness, never approached
by him before or afterwards. All doubt of his insanity
was now removed in the judgment of his physician.
That judgment was afterward fully confirmed, by a
complete developement of the disease.

As there is disease of intellect, without disease of
the passions, so there may be disease of the passions,
without apparent disease of intellect.* In diseases of
the pathetical states or functions, there may be *exaltation* or *depression* of one or more of the passions.
These diseases are more to be dreaded than any
others, to which man is liable. The passions, being
the source of all his actions, and continually demand-
ing of the intellectual powers the means of their
gratification, if they be in excess, they urge to action
beyond the bounds of reason, and the subject of them
is driven and hurried on to the perpetration of the
most atrocious deeds. Here the law sees no delusion,
and holds the miserable offender accountable for his
acts. This, perhaps, is the only practicable rule, consistent with the safety of society.

The physician, however, must take a different view
of these deplorable cases. He must discard the
policy of the law, and attend to the voice of humanity
and of truth. It is true, the passions are under the
control of every man in a state of sound mind. Whoever possesses this power of control, and neglects to

* Pinel. Manie sans délire. § 64.

exercise it, is responsible for deeds arising from his negligence. But the man, who has lost this power by the *exaltation* of one or more of the passions, who does not possess that self-control, which belongs to every man of sound mind, labors under a mental *defect*,—a deviation, which as truly constitutes a disease, as does any deviation from a state of health in the intellectual or vital functions. If the passions are all in due proportion, they are productive of the good, for which our Creator designed them. But when one or more of them is exalted, they will be followed by mental disturbance. Such may be their influence upon the intellectual powers, that what is right, or what is wrong may not be discerned ; or the feeling of obligation to avoid the latter and pursue the former may be overpowered, or lost in the *diseased desire* of gratification. There may be an extravagance of feeling, as there was in the days of chivalry, or the crusades, or has been in periods of religious or political excitement, which may obscure the intellectual vision, and lead the blinded enthusiast into the greatest absurdities.

But there is another state of mind, in which one or more of the passions are *depressed*, and evince a defect of vigor and activity. There are persons, who are almost destitute of friendship, love, or hope, and nearly all the kind and benevolent affections. Others are scarcely susceptible of hatred, envy, or revenge, &c. And again, there are some, in whom there is a kind of general apathy, who feel no interest in the affairs of life, or in the happiness of themselves or of others. These are deviations from a sound state, and fall within the conditions of mental disease. They are not the natural and original states of the individual, but temporary changes induced by particular causes.

Exaltation, and depression of passion, are sometimes manifested alternately in the same individual. * * has been for several years subject to alternations of these states, without disease of the intellectual powers. During the state of depression he talks little—scarcely answers questions—goes to bed early—sleeps well—rises late—takes food regularly—is indifferent about his dress—refuses to walk, or ride, or to attend church —writes no letters—reads no newspapers—discovers no interest in any person or kind of business. He is not anxious, or distressed on any subject—is perfectly quiet and inoffensive. After being depressed from two to five weeks, he gradually becomes more active, gay, and full of business. As a first change, he begins to smile, and answer questions ; then to sit up later, sleep less and rise earlier—walks, and rides when requested. In a few days, he begins to converse freely, read newspapers, and play at chess. Next he calls for his best clothes —is anxious to attend church, visit every where, and see every body—plans voyages—is full of business—writes letters to all parts of the United States, to England, France, Holland, &c.—becomes gay—dances, sings—is irrascible—offended when opposed—passionate, and violent—tears his clothes—breaks windows, swears, strikes, kicks, bites, dashes drinks in the faces of attendants, and sometimes says, ' I would send you to hell, if I could ; ' but instantly, sensible of the inhumanity of his wishes, and becoming calm, adds, with good feeling, 'But I would remove you to heaven in one minute.' The paroxysms of passion, in various degrees, are repeated many times in a day, from the most trifling causes, and without malice. In this case, the changes from depression to exaltation of passion are usually gradual—often sudden, and sometimes instantaneous. The paroxysms are, almost universally, free from any apparent disease of the intellectual powers. His letters are well written, his plans of voyages are judicious, and the whole discovers an intimate knowledge of business. When the transitions are gradual, he appears, during the intervals, quite well for several weeks, and is a kind hearted, intelligent, agreeable man.

To exhibit clear and exact views of an insane mind, it seemed necessary to consider separately diseases of the intellect, and diseases of the passions ; yet they are seldom so observed in fact. During health the intellect may discover some supposed good, real or imaginary, and then will arise the desire to obtain it ; or it may detect some supposed evil, real or imaginary, and then will arise the desire to avoid it, and, perhaps, to punish its author. Or one or more of the passions may become excited, and seek to be gratified, and then the intellect is to devise the means to accomplish the end. These relations continue in a state of *disease*, the disordered intellect suggesting opportunities for the indulgence of the passions, or the excited passions, in their turn, prompting the intellect to provide for their gratification. Hence the most common form of insanity is a combination of disordered passions, and disordered intellect, in variety and gradations almost infinite.

Such, too, is the connexion between the mental operations and various organic functions, that diseases of the one frequently induce diseases of the other. Hence insanity arising from moral causes, as jealousy, anger, remorse, unexpected adversity or prosperity, soon produces disease in some of the abdominal viscera. Hence, too, diseases of the alimentary tube, the liver, and the uterus, often produce mental diseases.

It has been my object to notice some of the connexions between sound mind and mental disease, that I might suggest for your future consideration the importance of mental philosophy, as a necessary part of a medical education. It is the number and extent of the mental powers of man, that constitutes the vast difference between him and every other terrestrial being. It is mind, that traverses the ocean, and converts a wilderness into fruitful fields. It was the mind of Newton, which explored the heavens, weighed the planets, and measured their distances. It was the mind of La Place, which again journeyed through the celestial regions, and returned with new proofs of the power and wisdom of the creator. But in the most exalted views of the mind of man, there appears enough of frailty to teach him humility. It is subject to disease. Its powers may be prostrated in a few uneasy days. In a single moment, the noblest intellect may be reduced to the humble condition of the most ordinary mind. Such changes are obvious to all, and leave no one in doubt of their nature. It it not usual, however, that the subversion of the mind is the work of an hour, or a day. The attacks of insanity are commonly gradual, and in passing from a state of sound mind to a state of derangement, the changes are almost imperceptible.

' Such thin partitions do the bounds divide,' that it may be difficult to form a satisfactory opinion, whether an individual be, or be not deranged. In determining a question so important to him, the first inquiry should certainly be to ascertain the actual states of mind, as manifested by the countenance, conversation, and conduct. But this knowledge will be of little use, unless it be compared with some standard—the standard of sound mind.

The medical student is required to learn of chemistry and natural philosophy the laws of inanimate matter—to toil, at the risk of life, in learning the structure of the body, and the functions of its organs ; yet it is only *incidentally*, that the functions of the mind become an object of his attention. That, which acquires all knowledge, may itself remain unknown. A knowledge of the faculties of the human mind, and the laws of its operations, can be acquired by no man except by deep attention to the mental changes, of which he is conscious. He must find within himself the facts and experiments, from which alone he can deduce the principles of mental science. In making these deductions, he will discover a new world, beautiful and wonderful, 'the image of God.'

Mental philosophy is interesting to physicians, as men of science. It will repay their labors, as curious men, seeking amusement ; as students of nature, of good morals, and of sound religion. It is also inter-

esting to them as a profession.   No where does it cast
a clearer or a stronger light, than it throws upon the
darkness of a disordered mind.   In cases of alleged
or pretended insanity, physicians are frequently called
to give opinions, upon which the verdict of a jury or
the judgment of a court may mainly depend.   Here
rests upon the medical witness a most solemn responsibility.   The decision may involve consequences, more
important to individuals and the community, than the
treatment of the disease.   It may extend to the disposition of property, validity of contracts, responsibility for crimes, even to the jeopardy of life.   Before
another anniversary of this society, some of its fellows
may be involved in a calamity, by which property, or
character, or life, may turn upon the question of
sanity or insanity.   It may be that this question will
be decided upon testimony, which some of you may
be required to give—and the correctness of this testimony may depend upon a correct knowledge of
sound mind.

NOTE A.—PAGE 6.

So various are the classifications of the functions of animated beings,
that it is impossible to speak of them intelligibly without some explanation.
In the preceding discourse the following arrangement has been observed.

VITAL FUNCTIONS—functions of living or animated beings.
    I. ORGANIC FUNCTIONS—functions of all organs, whether of
                vegetables or of animals.
    II. MENTAL FUNCTIONS—all mental changes or states; as
                knowing or being conscious.
                Intellectual—perceiving, remembering, &c.
                Pathetical—joy, grief—hope, fear—love, hatred,
                  &c.

1. Remark. Vegetables have only organic functions. Animals have
both organic and mental functions.

2. Remark. It must be obvious to every man, who attends to his
thoughts, that *knowledge* or *consciousness*, arising from changes in the
material world, is totally different from the changes, *from* which it arises.
They are followed by the state of being conscious, and are, in a certain
sense, the causes of that state.

3. Remark. The modern doctrine of two lives in one being, is not more simple, than the old doctrine of one being, composed of a living body and a thinking soul. The distinction between the organs of '*animal life*' and of '*organic life*,' as stated by Bichat, does not seem to be well founded. Of the former he considers the organs to be double, possessing 'symmetry of external forms ;' of the latter to be single, having 'irregularity of external forms.' The following enumeration of double and of single organs will show, that the distinction, as contended for, does not exist in man.

I. Organs, which are double, consisting of two analogous parts, viz.

The brain and nearly all the nerves—the eyes, ears and nostrils—the tongue and chin, divided by a medial line—the fingers and toes of one side, corresponding with those of the other—the lungs, heart, and nearly all the arteries and veins—the kidneys and ureters, united in the bladder—the prostrate gland—the testicles, vasa defferentia and vesiculæ seminales—the ovaria and fallopian tubes, united in the uterus—the parotid, submaxillary, axillary and inguinal glands—nearly all the bones and muscles.

II. Organs, which are single, viz. the œsophagus, stomach, intestines, liver, pancreas and spleen. Perhaps the uterus and bladder may be considered either as single organs, or as the union and continuation of double organs.

Note B.—Page 10.

The treatment of insanity chiefly depends upon the connexion between the mind and body. If there be inflammation of the brain, or its membranes, it is to be treated as inflammation of those parts. If there be other organic disease, whether of structure or of function, in any part of the body, medical treatment will be required. But in mental disorders, without symptoms of organic disease, a judicious moral management is more successful. It should afford agreeable occupation. It should engage the mind, and exercise the body ; as swinging, riding, walking, sewing, embroidery, bowling, gardening, mechanic arts ; to which may be added reading, writing, conversation, &c. the whole to be performed with order and regularity. Even the taking of food, retiring to bed, rising in the morning, &c. at stated times, and conforming to stated rules in almost everything, is a most salutary discipline. It requires, however, constant attention and vigilance, with the greatest kindness and attention in the attendants upon a lunatic. Moral treatment is indispensable, even in cases arising from organic disease.

In regard to medical treatment, I believe, that purging, bleeding, low diet, &c. have been adopted with little discrimination. They are to be resorted to only when there is organic disease, which requires the '*reducing plan*.' But these remedies, especially in debilitated subjects, are seldom useful in relieving mental disease. They are usually injurious, and frequently fatal. It is undoubtedly true, that impressions upon the alimentary canal by purging or vomiting; and upon the skin of the extremities by blistering, are useful in chronic cases of mental disorders. But these remedies must be suited to the strength and general health of the patient.

AN

INAUGURAL DISSERTATION

ON

INSANITY:

SUBMITTED TO THE PUBLIC EXAMINATION OF THE TRUSTEES
OF THE COLLEGE OF PHYSICIANS AND SURGEONS,
IN THE STATE OF NEW-YORK,

SAMUEL BARD, M. D. PRESIDENT,

FOR THE DEGREE OF

DOCTOR OF MEDICINE,

ON THE 14TH DAY OF MAY, 1811.

BY THEODRIC ROMEYN BECK, A. M.

LICENTIATE IN MEDICINE OF THE MEDICAL SOCIETY OF THE
COUNTY OF NEW-YORK.

Canst thou not minister to a mind diseas'd ;
Pluck from the memory a rooted sorrow ;
Raze out the written troubles of the brain ;
And with some sweet oblivious antidote,
Cleanse the foul bosom of that perilous stuff,
Which weighs upon the heart ?　　MACBETH

NEW-YORK :
PRINTED BY J. SEYMOUR, No. 49, JOHN-STREET.

1811.

TO THE

REV. JOHN B. ROMEYN, D. D.

THIS DISSERTATION

IS MOST SINCERELY INSCRIBED,

WITH ALL THE FEELINGS

THAT GRATITUDE, ESTEEM, AND THE HIGHEST RESPECT

CAN INSPIRE,

BY HIS AFFECTIONATE NEPHEW,

THE AUTHOR.

INAUGURAL DISSERTATION

INSANITY.

——————

"Of the uncertainties of our present state," says Dr. Johnson, " the most dreadful and alarming is, the uncertain continuance of reason." The sage was himself a mournful example of what melancholy, and the fear of the loss of reason, could effect in a mind at once original, capacious, and powerful. Indeed, men of genius and talents seem, in many instances, to fall victims to the disease of insanity. It embittered the life of Cowper; shrouded in mental darkness the declining days of Swift; and prostrated the acute understanding of Vicq. D'Azyr. This spectacle of " human nature in ruins," which, while it attacks the learned and wise, does not spare those engaged in other pursuits, has attracted the attention of medical men and philosophers in all ages and countries. Their examinations have thrown light on a mysterious subject, but much remains to be still unfolded. A compilation of the more important facts contained in their writings, relative to this disease, is all that can be expected from one whose opportunities of viewing the disease have been scanty, and whose information is derived chiefly from books.

B

10

The most common, and probably the most accurate division of the faculties and powers of the mind, is that into *understanding* and *will*. Under the former are included *perception*, or the impression made by external objects on the organs of sense, the nerves, and the brain, and conveyed, by means of consciousness, to the mind; *memory*, comprehending both a power of retaining knowledge, and of recalling it to our thoughts when occasion requires; *judgment* and *reason*, or the faculty of discerning the relation of one thought or proposition with another, and drawing inferences from them; and *imagination*, whose province it is to make a selection of qualities and circumstances from various sources, and by combining and disposing them, to form a new creation of its own. To these may be added, *attention*, *abstraction*, and *conception*. The will comprehends the active powers, as the *passions* and *affections*. In most, if not in all the operations of the mind, both these faculties concur. Perception is one that arrives to maturity, even in infancy. The impressions of external objects are the first which occur to the view, and consequently claim the greatest share of regard. The rest are developed and improved with advancing years. Memory, assisted by attention*, treasures up the knowledge which we have acquired; whilst reason, in a well governed mind, always exercises a commanding sway over the imagination and passions, regulating the excursions of the one, and restraining the excesses of the other†.

* " Attention to things external is properly called *observation*; and attention to the subjects of our consciousness, *reflection*."—REID.
† Vide Reid and Stewart.

These faculties are, however, far from being uniform in all men. They are influenced, amongst a
variety of other causes, by early education, habit,
improper association of ideas, and differences in the
physical constitution. Through the varied operation
of these agents, our actions in life are guided, and according as they differ from the standard which the
general sense of mankind has adopted, are regarded
as deviations from sanity or virtue. The diseases of
the mind included under the former are numerous,
and have been called by various names. It will probably simplify our remarks on them, by sketching
those of the more important faculties separately. *Perception* is liable to injury, both in itself and in its
immediate órgans. The senses may be affected in
numberless ways, by bodily disease. The power
itself becomes erroneous, from ignorance, and other
subordinate causes, as rashness and credulity. Objects are also at different times presented in too great
rapidity, or too slowly, producing the different states
of *vertigo* and *ennui*. To this class may also be
referred the belief in the appearance of apparitions*.
It appears to be altogether destroyed, or at least very
seldom brought into operation, in fatuity or idiotism,
in which " no accurate representation of any external object, and no abstract thought or reflection ever
occurs†." The *memory* may be injured by various

* Vide an interesting paper " on Apparitions, by John
Alderson, M. D." in Edin. Med. and Surg. Journal, vol. vi.
p. 287. The author discusses this diseased state of perception, and establishes the difference between it, and læsions of
other faculties, in a rational and conclusive manner.
† Crichton on Mental Derangement, vol. 1. p. 314.

corporeal agents, for which I need only refer to the writings of practical physicians. It decays in old age, and among the mental causes which affect it, are to be included inattention and over-exertion. It is a remarkable fact, that persons advanced in life remember the scenes of youth much better than the transactions of later years. The same thing has occurred in cases of old, incurable lunatics*. The *judgment* and *reason*, the peculiar birthright of man, become erroneous, defective, or are totally destroyed. Prejudice, passion, ignorance, and all the agents which affect the other faculties, assist in weakening it. Among the disorders of the *imagination*, may be mentioned reverie, or the illusion of waking dreams, and too great sensibility. The latter is the fruitful source of ills, producing enthusiasm, fastidious refinement, and inattention to the necessary business of life. The consequences of ill-regulated *passions* need not to be mentioned. The other powers are subject to similar imperfections. All of them are more or less disordered in mental derangement, but which of them primarily, is difficult to be determined.

An an logy has been supposed by some to exist between the states of dreaming and insanity, and the opinion has some foundation; particularly if Prof. Stewart's theory be correct, viz. that the power of the will is suspended during sleep†. Dreams, according to him, vary with our bodily sensations, the prevailing temper of mind, and our habits of association, when awake. The distinction of Haslam, which is

* Haslam on Madness, &c. 2d edit. p. 61.

† It will, however, be difficult to account for somnambulism, and talking in sleep, on this supposition.

borrowed from Hartley, that in madness the delusion is conveyed principally through the ear, while in dreaming it is optical, will hardly stand the test of fact. A remarkable instance to the contrary is related by Dr. Beattie, in his Dissertation on Dreaming.

From the foregoing imperfect sketch of the " Anatomy of the mind," it will be seen that it is subject to disease as well as the body. To arrange the various kinds according to their proper gradations, is almost impossible in the present imperfect state of this science. The following comprehends most of those concerning which we have information. Pleasant dreams*, unpleasant dreams, somnambulism, vigilia, erroneousness of judgment in children, dotage of old

* Although it will not be denied, that unpleasant dreams are a state of disease, yet many may not be disposed to allow the same concerning pleasant ones. Several circumstances, however, tend to substantiate this assertion, such as the necessity of rest to the mind, as well as the body, the disordered state of the imagination during sleep, unswayed by judgment, and the fact of persons, who are in habits of thinking, and thus causing over-activity of the mind, dreaming much, while the contrary description of persons, as the labourer, do not. Locke, (Essay, book 2. chap. 1.) mentions the case of a gentleman who never dreamt, till he had a fever in the 25th year of his age. Dr. Beattie, (Dissert. on Dreaming,) mentions a person who never dreamt but when his health was disordered. Medical men have made similar observations. " Observamus somnum, qui ante mediam noctem. capitur, plus incrementi viribus addere, quam qui eam subsequitur. Ratio hæc esse videtur, quia, homines tunc temporis profundiori somno merguntur." Hoffman. Opera Fol. Tom. 1. p. 126. An. 1748. Gregory, (Conspectus, vol. 1. p. 209.) remarks, " Qui sanissimi altum dormiunt, iis neque motus voluntarius est, neque sensus externus, neque interni, si quis fuerit, ulla memoria."

age, reverie, too great liveliness of imagination, disordered association of ideas, frequent recurrence of
the same train of thought, loss of memory, nervous
affections, violent passions, hypochondriasis, hysteria,
epilepsy, madness, melancholy, fatuity, together with
delirium, and other affections attendant on acute dis-
tempers. Many of these, if not all, are connected
with diseases of the body,

—◦◦—

HISTORY OF THE DISEASE.

IN the earliest medical writings of the ancients,
insanity is divided into melancholia and mania. Although Hippocrates has left us no particular treatise
on this subject, yet it is clearly deducible from various parts of his works, that he considered them as
different forms oi disease*. Aretœus, the first writer
extant who treats professedly on diseases of the mind,
adopts this distinction, but observes, that melancholy
appears to him to be the commencement, and constitutes part of mania†; and succeeding writers, with
hardly an exception, have followed this arrangement,
until within the last twenty years. Several systems
have been offered to the world‡, in which insanity is

* Compare Aphorisms, Sect. 3. Aphor. 20. and 22. and
Sect. 6. Aphor. 23. with Lib. De Morbo Sacro, Sect. 3. p. 92.
(Ed. Fœsii.)

† " Mihi profecto melancholia μανία;, initium atque pars
esse videtur." Aretæus De Caus Diut. affect. lib. 1. p. 29. Ed.
Boerhaave, 1735. Cælius Aurelianus observes, that Themi-
son and his disciples were of the same opinion. De Morb.
Chron. lib. 1. 340. Ed. Amman.

‡ By Drs. Arnold, Crichton, and Pincl.

divided into a number of species; but they have generally been found as useless in practice, as they are
difficult to be distinguished in theory. The idea of
their being one and the same disease, in different
forms, according to the temperament and constitution
of the patient, seems not unreasonable. The facts
of the very frequent conversion of one into the other;
of numbers whose lives are passed between furious
and melancholic paroxysms, and under both, retaining
the same set of ideas* ; and of the same remedies,
with little variation, being found useful for both, materially strengthen this supposition. Mr. Haslam,
whose opportunities of viewing the disease in all its
varied forms, have been very great, observes, " In
both there is equal derangement, and on dissection,
the state of the brain does not show any appearances
peculiar to melancholia†." As, however, the symptoms which are immediately presented to our view
appear so diametrically opposite, it will be proper to
retain the distinction. Insanity may be divided into
melancholy, mania, and *idiotism.* The first is cha-
racterised by an anxious look, love of solitude, and
excess of fear. The second by hurried action, lo-
quacity, and furious raving. The last, although frequently the termination of the previous ones, is in
many instances an idiopathic disease‡. Its peculiar
character has been already noticed.

Various theories have been proposed, as it respects
the affection of the mind in these stages. In melancholy it is invariably fixed on a single train of

* Haslam on Madness, p. 33.
† Haslam, p. 37.
‡ As in the Cretins of Switzerland.

thought*: while in mania, it is roving with rapidity from one subject to another. By an application of the principles already laid down, the difficulty of arriving at any certainty on this point will be immediately perceived. Maniacs, in many instances, have false perceptions; that is, they assert they have seen objects which it is impossible could have appeared to them. But this defect is not universal. In some the idea is evidently derived from former impressions, and no trace can be perceived of diseased perception. The reasoning faculty also, though impaired, is not destroyed. The patient argues correctly from false premises. We are ignorant of the train of thought passing in his mind, and judge only by the incoherence of his conversation, which may be owing to the rapidity of his ideas, and his expressing only part of them. The ideas may be represented either with *unnatural rapidity*, *unnatural association*, or *unnatural vividness*†. The passions appear occasionally to be the seat of insanity, unaccompanied with defect of judgment and imagination. The whole disease in this case appears to consist in a preternatural susceptibility to emotions. It may be said, that these different læsions of the faculties of the mind certainly prove the existence of different diseases; but the objection is at once repelled by the fact of a single patient at various times passing through all the gradations, from furious phrenzy to complete fatuity.

---

* " Est autem (in melancholia) animi angor in una cogitatione defixus." Aretæus ut antea. Dr. Ferriar's definition of melancholy is, " intensity of idea," *granting an object exclusive attention.*

† London Med. Review, vol. 1. p. 46.

patients from their residence to some proper asylum; and for this purpose, a calm retreat in the country is to be preferred: for it is found that continuance at home aggravates the disease, as the improper association of ideas cannot be destroyed. A system of humane vigilance is adopted. Coercion, by blows, stripes, and chains, although sanctioned by the authority of Celsus and Cullen, is now justly laid aside. The rules most proper to be observed are the following: Convince the lunatics that the power of the physician and keeper is absolute; have humane attendants, who shall act as servants to them; never threaten but execute; offer no indignities to them, as they have a high sense of honour; punish disobedience peremptorily, in the presence of the other maniacs: if unruly, forbid them the company of others, use the strait waistcoat, confine them in a dark and quiet room, order spare diet, and if danger is apprehended, apply metallic manacles to their hands and feet, as they are found not to injure by friction so much as linen or cotton; tolerate noisy ejaculations; strictly exclude visitors; let their fears and resentments be soothed without unnecessary opposition; adopt a system of regularity; make them rise, take exercise and food at stated times. The diet ought to be light, and easy of digestion, but never too low. When convalescent, allow limited liberty; introduce entertaining books and conversation, exhilirating music, employment of body in agricultural pursuits, as is the case in the hospitals of York and Saragossa; and admit friends under proper restrictions. It will also be proper to forbid their returning home too soon. By thus acting, the patient will " minister to himself."

The following is the most correct explanation, (though liable to objection,) which the author has met with, and is one that will elucidate a great number of the phænomena that occur. " The true relation between the two general forms of insanity may be stated to consist in *abstraction*, and in *vivid imagination*. The one will comprehend that state, where the mind separates the combinations which are presented to it, and fixes its attention exclusively upon one single object. The other combines the different objects and various sensations, creates new ones, and mistakes conceptions, the recollection of past perceptions for real existences.*"

A similar diversity of opinion has taken place, (though not in so great a degree,) as to its seat in the body. Hippocrates supposed the brain to be affected in two ways, by the bile and pituita; the heating and cooling principle. The one causing mania, and the other melancholy†. Aurelianus supposed the head to be disordered in the former, and the stomach in the latter‡. The moderns in general refer it to the brain, allowing, however, in some instances, that the stomach is the primary organ diseased. A kind of

* Edinburgh Review, vol. 2. p. 169.

† " At cerebri corruptio ex pituita et bile oritur, utrumque autem hoc modo dignosces. Qui ex pituita quidem insaniunt, quieti sunt, neque vociferantur, neque tumultuantur; qui vero ex bile, clamosi, maligni et minime quieti, semper aliquid intempestivum faciunt. Ex his igitur causis continuo insaniunt." De Morbo Sacro Sect. 3. p. 92. line 36. (Ed. Foesii)

‡ " Differt autem, siquidem in ista (melancholia) principaliter stomachus patitur, in furiosis vero caput." Cæl. Aurelian. ut antea.

chronic inflammation or plethora of the vessels of the brains, supposed by many to occur. In what the other changes from health consist, it is difficult to explain.

The *diagnosis*, or distinguishing symptom of insanity, has been universally stated to be " *delirium sine febre.*" The correctness of this is destroyed, by the fact, of a patient during the hysteric paroxysms being in the same situation.

The difficulty of giving a correct *definition*, has been of late unwillingly acknowledged. " There is, indeed, a double difficulty ; the definition ought to comprehend the aberrations of the lunatic, and fix the standard of the practitioner. But it may be assumed, that sound mind and insanity stand in the same predicament, and are opposed to each other in the same manner as right and wrong, and as truth to the lie*."

—◦◦◦—

SYMPTOMS.

IN many instances, an attack of insanity is preceded by pain in the head, throbbing of the arteries, and even giddiness; tightness about the region of the abdomen, want of appetite, peculiar sensation in the intestines, costiveness, loss of sleep. All the patients agree that they feel confused from the sudden and rapid intrusion of unconnected thoughts.

They who are attacked with *mania* become uneasy; are unable to confine their attention ; are loquacious ; walk with a quick and hurried step, and stop suddenly. They express their opinions with great fervency and extravagance, and are highly impatient

* Haslam, p. 37.

of reproof. Some laugh, cry, and sing, by turns.
The eyes protrude, and are often glistening. The
cheeks are flushed. A relaxation of the integuments
of the occiput, together with contraction of the iris,
occur in some cases. A very vigorous action of
both body and mind takes place, particularly great
muscular strength. Some fancy themselves kings,
prophets, &c. Some feel an ungovernable inclination to acts of fury and violence, and maim and
murder those whom they can approach. They become suspicious of plots. This fury increases, until
at last confinement is necessary ; while in that situation they are observed to continue a particular action
for a length of time, such as shaking their chains, or
beating with their feet. They readily yield to superior force, and a stern countenance.

The *melancholic* attack, on the other hand, com-
mences with a gloomy, anxious countenance ; little
disposition to speak; avoidance of company, frequently keeping the eye " bent on vacuity," for hours.
The patient often bursts into tears ; imagines he has
committed some heinous crime, and not unfrequently
finishes his hated existence.

The maniac and melancholic, however, do not always remain in these situations; the paroxysms abate,
and are succeeded by calmness, and a certain degree
of rationality. This has been called the *lucid interval.*
" I have no where," says Pinel, " met, excepting in
romances, with fonder husbands, more affectionate parents, more impassioned lovers, *more pure and exalted
patriots,* than in the lunatic asylum, during the intervals of calmness and reason*. Its duration is, how-

* Pinel on Insanity, translated by Dr. Davis, p, 16.

ever, very uncertain, and ought to have no weight with the physician, as to preventing watchfulness, and pursuing the proper method of cure. The exhaustion that follows the paroxysm is highly dangerous, and must be carefully guarded against*.

Madmen are said to possess the *power of resisting cold;* but this is denied by late writers. Mr. Haslam observes, that they are very subject to mortification of the toes from exposure to inclement weather†. Those that are permitted to walk about are always found near the fire in winter. Probably the great engagement of the mind causes insensibility during the paroxysm. They are also said to possess the *power of resisting hunger.* Many refuse food, from an apprehension of being poisoned. In some instances the fasting has been prolonged to fourteen days‡. Mr. Pinel gives a melancholy account of the mortality in the Asylums of France, during the storms of the revolution, when the daily allowance of bread was reduced§.

Of the organs of sense the ear is most affected ; many become deaf, but very few blind‖. The majority of patients grow worse from lying in the recumbent posture. Of 265 lunatics, in Bethlem hospital, who were examined, 205 were swarthy, with dark or black

* Haslam, Pinel, and Ferriar. " Whoever," says the latter, " would gain a knowledge of the symptoms of madness from books, more particularly than that afforded by Aretæus, must consult *Shakspeare.*" In proof of this I need only refer to the tragedies of *Lear, Macbeth,* and *Hamlet.*

† P. 84.

‡ Annals of Medicine, vol. 5. p. 383.

§ Pinel, p. 33. and 209.

‖ Haslam, p. 67.

hair, and 60 with fair skin, and light, brown, and red haired*. It is a remark made by Hoffman, and confirm- ed by experience, that maniacs are not subject to epi- demics. Dr. Hosack informs me, that none were at- tacked with yellow fever during its prevalence in this city. Other diseases are also removed by its at- tack†.

The appearance of *idiots* are marked by looks de- void of animation, and motion slow and mechan- ical. The senses are imperfectly developed, and the train of ideas, (if any exist,) are very slow and fee- ble. Many of them, after remaining in this state for years, are attacked with paroxysms of active mania, and the symptom is favourable, since in some cases it is succeeded by a return of reason‡. Congenite idiotism is found in the Vallais in Switzerland, in Sa- voy, in the island of Sumatra, in Chinese Tartary, near the great wall, as observed by Sir George Staun- ton§. In most cases they are affected with goitre. A diminution of the size of the cranium, as well as of the brain, is also said to occur‖. This interesting subject

* Haslam, p. 83. " Novimus enim hirsutos, nigroque colo- re et habitu tenues, multo facilius quam candidos et cras- siores, melancholia corripi." Alex. Trallian, voi. 1. p. 84. (Ed. Haller, 1772.)

† Vide Mead's Med. Precepts, and Ferriar on the Con- version of Diseases.

‡ Pinel, p. 168.

§ Coxe's Travels in Switzerland, 4th edit. vol. 1. p. 420. et Seq.

‖ In a Lecture on Physiology, delivered at Paris, by Dr. Gall, Jan. 15, 1808, he stated as his opinion, that the power of intelligence was in proportion to the developement of the brain. Thus stupid animals have very little brain, sagacious

is further elucidated in Fodéré " Essai sur le Goitre et Cretenisme," and in Dr. Reeve's " Account of Cretenism," in Edin. Med. & Surg. Journal, vol. 5. p. 31.

CAUSES.

THE remote causes of insanity are either bodily or mental.

Bodily causes. Repeated intoxication ; blows, and other injuries on the head ; fever, particularly when attended with delirium ; cutaneous eruptions repelled ; suppression of periodical or occasional discharges and secretions ; excessive evacuations ; mercury largely and injudiciously administered* ; paralytic affections ; great heat of climate ; *coup de soleil;* changes of the moon† ; influence of the seasons, particularly summer‡ ; in England, the *month of November ;* hereditary predisposition ; melancholic, and probably the sanguineous temperament ; manufactures§.

ones more, none so much as man ; and among men idiots are remarkable for smallness of the head, and paucity of brain. He exhibited the heads of several idiots in proof of this position. Literary Panorama, vol. 4. p. 164.

* Haslam.

† Hence called lunatics. This cause, although denied by Haslam and others to be one, has the testimony of many physicians in favour of it, and among the rest may be named Dr. Balfour in his Theory of Sol Lunar Influence. Vide Asiatic Researches, vol. 8th.

‡ Pinel.

§ According to the Report of the Committee of the House of Commons, in 1807, Lancashire has 272 lunatics.

Mental causes. The principal source of these is, errors in *early education;* pursuing a system which injures the body, gives free scope to the passions, and does not discipline the intellect. It would be a highly interesting speculation, to consider, in connexion with this subject, the differences in the moral and physical constitution of man, produced by successive changes from barbarism to civilization; together with the influence of increase of wealth and luxury. National character deserves also to be noticed. England, Switzerland, and Spain, have the greatest number of lunatics, in proportion to their population, of any countries in Europe. In France there were but few, until the Revolution*. The frequent and uncurbed indulgence of any violent passions or emotions are the most common mental causes. Gray has delineated their effects with graphic accuracy.—

> These shall the fury passions tear,
> The *vultures* of the mind,
> Disdainful *anger*, pallid *fear*,
> And *shame* that skulks behind ;
> Or pining *love* shall waste their youth,
> Or *jealousy* with rankling tooth,
> That inly gnaws the secret heart,
> And *envy* wan, and faded *care*,
> Grim visag'd comfortless *despair*,
> And *sorrow's* piercing dart.

---

out of a population of 670,000, while the counties of Cambridge, Huntingdon, Hertford, and Essex, have 7, out of 444,000. The East Riding of Yorkshire three ; North Riding, twenty-three ; while the West Riding has 424. Literary Panorama, vol. 2. p. 1259.

* Arnold on Insanity, vol. 1. sect. 2.

Ambition this shall tempt to rise,
Then whirl the wretch from high,
To bitter scorn a sacrifice,
And grinning infamy.

Avarice, domestic misfortunes, commercial specu-
lations*, political contests†, *enthusiastic patriotism‡*,
mistaken ideas of religion causing either enthusiasm
or superstition, and sudden joy, may also be mentioned. Minds destitute of order in their intellectual
operations, are much predisposed to insanity.

Of 113 madmen confined at Bicetre, in 1795, Mr.
Pinel found, that 34 were reduced to that state by
domestic misfortunes, 24 by disappointments in love,
30 by events connected with the Revolution, and 25
by religious fanaticism. The subjects were principally monks, many artists, painters, and musicians,
versifiers, " who have all the melancholy madness of
poetry, without its inspiration ;" and a great number
of *advocates* and *attornies*. No instances of a single
physician, chemist, or mathematician§.

Of the *Proximate Cause* we know nothing.

———•———

DISSECTIONS.

IT is well observed by Dr. Arnold, that in no
disease are the appearances on dissection more falla-
cious, as to guiding us in our opinion of the seat and
cause of it, than in insanity. According to him

* Willan.
† Rush.
‡ Pinel, p. 15.
§ Pinel, p. 113, 114

this must be attributed to the danger of mistaking effects for causes. The following are among the more remarkable appearances of the brain, which occurred in the dissections of Morgagni, Greding*, and Haslam. The dura and pia mater diseased, and water between them. The consistence of the brain in most instances soft, in some cases quite elastic†. Pineal gland diseased. Water in the ventricles. Hydatids on the plexus choroides. Vessels of the brain distended, and the brain itself showing marks of inflammation or congestion. In slight cases, nothing particular was observed, except a determination of blood. Nothing important was observed in the viscera. M. Prost, a physician in Paris, places insanity in the stomach and bowels, as he has found the intestines and gall bladder diseased in several dissections of maniacs‡. Mr. Pinel supposes, that in the majority of cases there is no organic læsion of the brain, on account of the success which attended the exclusive use of moral management§.

PROGNOSIS.

Sex. By a reference to the Appendix, it will be seen, that in England females are more liable to this complaint than men ; whilst on the continent the contrary takes place‖.

* Medical Aphorisms, translated by Crichton.
† Haslam, chap. 3.
‡ Edin. Med. & Surg. Journal, vol. 1. p. 455.
§ Pinel, p. 5.
‖ " Viri sane et furore et melancholia corripiuntur ; rarius autem quam viri, sed deterius mulieres furiis agitantur.

Age. By a similar examination it appears, that the number of patients admitted at Bethlem and Bicetre, between the age of 30 and 40, were greater, than between any other ten years. This is probably owing to the circumstances of misfortunes affecting the mind more sensibly at that time of life, when a family is generally to be provided for. Intoxication is also readily induced at that age, from similar causes; and the hereditary predisposition, (if any exists,) will make its appearance. Instances of insane children are rare. Mr. Haslam relates three cases, of the respective ages of three, seven, and ten years*.

State of Disease. Of 100 patients in a furious state, 62 were cured: of 100 melancholic, only 27†. If the disease arise from physical causes, the prognosis is more favourable than when from moral ones; thus, of 80 cases of puerperal mania, 50 recovered‡. The chance of cure is diminished in proportion to the length of time that the disease has remained. The frequent alternations of raving and melancholy madness are unfavourable, as are also those in which the temper is more affected than the understanding§. Heaviness after the paroxysm, hæmoptisis and cutaneous eruptions, are favourable symptoms. Relapses are frequent from affections of the mind, or error in diet and regimen. Madness, of the hereditary or religious

Ætas, quæ prope statum est, et ipse status huic malo subjiciuntur." Aretæus, Lib. 1. De Caus. Morb. Diutur. p. 30.

  * Haslam, chap. 4.

  † Haslam, p. 257.

  ‡ Haslam, p. 247.

  § Ferriar's Essay on Insanity, in Med. Hist. & Reflect. vol. 2.

kinds; or complicated with epilepsy and paralysis, or gradually declining into idiotism, is generally incurable. In addition to the statements in the appendix, it may be added, that Dr. Willis deposed, that of patients committed to him within three months after the attack, nine out of ten recovered; and Dr. Arnold states, that in his own private establishment, and the Leicester lunatic asylum, two thirds of those admitted are cured*. Dr. Rush is said to have cured twelve out of thirteen; and of recent cases cures four out of five†.

Termination. It is an observation of Celsus‡, and confirmed by succeeding writers, that insanity does not prevent patients from arriving at old age. Dr. Heberden attributes this to the parts of the brain, which are subservient to animal life, being distinct from those which are essential to the use of reason§. Lunatics are very subject to diarrhea. The diseases which generally close their unhappy existence are, apoplexy, palsy, phthisis, atrophy, and hydrothorax∥.

CURE.

AS the causes are of different kinds, so it is proper that the cure should be appropriate to each. For the removal of insanity arising from mental causes, a method is at present pursued, styled in general, MORAL MANAGEMENT. This consists in removing

---

* Quarterly Review, vol. 2. p. 160.
† This fact is communicated to the author by Prof. J. A. Smith.
‡ De Medicina, lib. 1. sect. 18. " Ut vitam non impediat."
§ Heberden's Med. Commentaries, p. 277.
∥ Greding.

REMEDIES. A comparison of the ancients with the moderns in this particular, will fully prove, that but few important improvements have been made by the latter. A general abstract of the practice of the most distinguished of each, is all that the length of this Dissertation will allow. Aretæus recommends moderate venæsection ; to be repeated, if the patient is plethoric, purging with black hellebore, and in some cases emetics ; nourishing diet. If arising from suppressed discharges, more active remedies are advised. He also mentions bathing in warm mineral waters, friction with oil, and purges exhibited occasionally for a length of time*. Trallian has similar directions ; he prefers topical bleeding, as it does not debilitate so much as venæsection. He also recommends the warm bath highly, and condemns the use of white hellebore, as a vomit, being too violent†. It is remarkable, that in the writings of the ancients, no traces are to be found of their considering hellebore as a specific, although this is the received opinion. It has probably arisen from the poet's enlarging on its virtues in a metaphorical manner. Aurelianus recommends shaving of the head, and the application of sinapisms‡. Celsus speaks in high terms of the use of cold water to the head§. Poppies applied to the head were advised by some, but it does not appear that they were generally used.

* Aretæus De Curat. Diut. Affect. lib. 1. chap. 5.

† Trallian, lib. 1. chap. 17.

‡ Aurelianus, De Morb. Chron. lib. 1. chap. 5 and 6. He rejects a remedy that had been advised by some, and gives the following reason : " Quippe cum sit possibile ex consuetis perficere sanitatem." P. 341.

§ Celsus, lib. 3. sect. 18.

Dr. Harvey's method of cure was by repeated bleedings, mild purges, and chalybeates†. Dr. Thomas Willis speaks in high terms of iron in melancholy‡. The practice of Hoffman is similar to the above. Dr. Mead, besides these remedies, advises attention to the evacuation by urine in cases of madness, and directs nitre to be used. He found blisters hurtful in most cases, and preferred setons in the neck. He also gave medicines to promote perspiration : ordered frequent use of the cold bath ; and in some instances prescribed anodynes§.

Among the practitioners of the last century and the present day, the method of cure of the following deserves notice. Dr. *Ferriar* found single emetics at the commencement of the disease useful, but objects to nauseating doses of tartrite of antimony frequently repeated, and gives cautions similar to the above named with respect to venæsection. He speaks in very high terms of the strict antiphlogistic treatment in cases arising from intemperance, but has found camphor, digitalis, and opium, even in large quantities, of no benefit. He uses the warm bath in mania, and the cold, together with bark and wine, in melancholy, with great advantage. Setons and blisters, were found beneficial. Under the head of purges, he prefers calomel, but. in several cases where he gave it so as to cause salivation, it pro-

† " De se testatur, quod aliquot maniacos per venæsectionem, bis vel ter repetitas, lenes purgationes et medicamenta antihypochondriaca mineralia, intra sex septimanas feliciter curaverit." De Vanitatibus, &c. Medicorum ; In Acta Eruditorum, 1701. p. 438.

‡ " De Anima Brutorum" in Opera, 1695. vol. 2. p. 278.

§ Mead's Medical Precepts and Cautions.

duced no sensible effect on the disease*. Mr. *Haslam* prefers blood drawn from the head by cupping, to any other method. He has found cathartics of great service. Jalap and senna are principally used. He found emetics and cold baths hurtful, in many cases inducing paralytic affections; and opium and setons useless. Blisters applied to the legs were advantageous, in some instances†. *Prof. Pinel* speaks slightingly of all kind of remedies, as he considers the disease to be curable by moral management alone. He recommends however a few drams of sulphate of magnesia, as an excellent preventive of approaching paroxysms‡. Dr. *Chiarugi*, of Florence, speaks in very high terms, of friction with opium ointment; it produced calmness in every case, and in some it affected a cure§. Dr. *Cox* uses the rotatory swing with similar success. Dr. *Rush* recommends venæsection to a large extent; mercury given so as to cause salivation; warm and cold bath; blisters to the ancles; together with fresh air and gentle exercise‖. The famous Dr. *Francis Willis*, who attended the present king of England, and the queen of Portugal, during their insanity, is said to have prefer-

* Medical Histories and Reflections, 1810. vol. 1. 214; and vol. 2. p. 107. In the Nova Acta Curios. vol. 1. p. 346. is related a case, cured by mercurial friction in a month, after all previous remedies had failed.

† Haslam, chap. 8. Dr. Hosack informs me, that he has found blisters applied to the head, and continued for a length of time, of great use.

‡ Page 44.

§ Annals of Medicine, vol. 3. p. 105.

‖ Med. Inquiries and Observations, 3d edit. vol. 4. p. 416.

& Coxe's Med. Muscum, vol. 4. p. 156.

red emetics. Opium he thought did harm; and when narcotics were required, he employed hyoscyamus. Blisters on the neck he found hurtful. Digitalis was considered proper in some cases, as was also the warm bath*. In the case of George III. which he attributed to weighty business, severe exercise, and too great abstemiousness; the bark, after a little calomel and a cathartic, appeared to be productive of very decided advantage†.

NOTE.—The Harvey, noticed above, was Dr. Gideon Harvey, physician to Charles II. in his exile. He flourished at the end of the seventeenth century.

MEDICAL JURISPRUDENCE AND POLICE.

THE Medical Jurisprudence of Lunatics may be considered in two points of view. 1. The security of the public, and 2. The proper treatment of the patients.

To effect the first, it becomes absolutely necessary that they should be confined in some convenient place, in order to prevent the commission of crimes, to which they are all more or less liable. The law has humanely forbidden the exercise of punishment on them, since its ends cannot be answered. " Society," (says Dr. Johnstone, and the sentiment is applauded by all good men,) " may obtain an adequate protection by the confinement of maniacs, without blood." Cases frequently occur, where medical men

* Edin. Med. & Surg. Journal, vol. 4. p. 195.
† Quarterly Review, vol. 2. p. 168.

are called on to decide before a jury respecting the state of a person's mind, who has committed a crime, or made an unjust will. In both, it is of importance, that they should have formed proper opinions on the several symptoms of this disease, for in none are men more apt to err, than on the apparent sanity of a maniac. The term *lucid interval* has been applied to this state. In matters of law, the following observation of Mr. Haslam is certainly the most proper to guide us : " I should define a *lucid interval* to be a complete recovery of the patient's intellects, ascertained by repeated examinations of his conversation, and by constant observation of his conduct, for a time sufficient to form a correct judgment*." Dr. Johnstone notices a discordance in the laws of England, which is highly disgraceful to a civilized nation. In matters of property, the law forbids the restoration of it, until the return of perfect reason and intellect, while merely appearances of sanity during the moment of committing a crime, are sufficient to condemn the maniac, although insane both before and after†. Whether this inhuman statute has force in our own country, the writer is unable to learn.‡

2. The *Treatment of Patients*. Different methods have been pursued for this purpose, according to the

* Haslam, p. 46.

† Medical Jurisprudence of Madness, by J. Johnstone, M. D. 1800.

‡ Dr. Mahon, in his Legal Medicine, observes, that in cases of maniacs committing crimes, we should follow the maxim of enlightened jurisconsults. " Semel furiosus, semper presumitur furiosus, et contrarium tenenti incumbit onus probandi sanam mentem." Lond, Med. & Phys. Journ. vol. 9. p. 72.

inclination of relatives, or the laws of the country. Thus criminal lunatics have been [confined in jails, but this is evidently incompatible with proper attendance, and the safety of the other prisoners. Nor is the plan of confinement in private mad-houses, free from objection. Even if their superintendants be humane, the accommodations are generally insufficient and inadequate for public security, since the instances of escape from them are numerous. But more important charges may be brought against them. They may be made, (and in Great-Britain are made,) the living tombs of the victims of avarice and revenge. In them the most dreadful cruelty may be exercised with impunity. To feel the justice of these censures, it is only necessary for any person to ask himself the question, What would be his feelings, were a relative or friend secluded in these abodes, through the malice of others? If private mad-houses are tolerated, they ought certainly to be watched with a jealous eye. The establishment of asylums, in various central parts of a country, exclusively appropriated to this purpose, under the particular superintendance of government, and open to the watchful inspection of proper commissioners, together with the advice and care of able physicians and humane keepers, is the plan which is open to the least objection, and is one which promises the happiest results as to the recovery and restoration of the insane to society *.

* Much interesting information on this subject will be found in the Report of the Committee of the house of Commons, and Prof. Duncan's paper on the State of Lunatics in Great-Britain, in Edin. Med. & Surg. Journal, vol. 4. p. 129, and 144.

APPENDIX.

THE following account of Lunatic Asylums in Europe and America, may probably be interesting to the reader.

ENGLAND.

THE largest establishments in England which are appropriated to the confinement of Lunatics are, St. Luke's and Bethlem Hospitals in London.

St. Luke's Hospital. This institution was founded in 1732, and opened in 1737. It then admitted 110 patients. On account of the increasing number of applicants, a new building, larger, and more commodious, was erected, in 1787, which accommodates 300 patients, divided into two lists or classes; 200 on the curable, and 100 on the incurable list. The latter are received according to the order in which they have been discharged as uncured from the Hospital. Of these there are at present (1810) more than 600 waiting for admission. Idiots are not admitted. Among its officers are, the Duke of Leeds President, and Dr. S. F. Simmons, Physician. The patients admitted from July 30, 1751, to April 21, 1809, amount to 9042, of which those discharged as incurable, and received again, amount to 323. Of these,

Patients remaining, April 21st. 1809,	-	-	-	199
discharged cured,	-	-	-	3915
uncured,	-	-	-	3101
as idiots,	-	-	-	783
dead,	- - -	-	-	748
taken away by friends, and discharged from various causes,	-	-	-	296
	-	-		9042

Patients received the second time, and remaining in the house,	-	-	-	100
taken away by friends,	-	-	-	56
dead,	-	-	-	145
cured,	-	-	-	18
discharged from various causes,		-	-	4
				323

Mr. Dunstan, Master of St. Luke's Hospital, states, in his examination before the Committee of the House of Commons, that the average number of curable patients admitted annually are, and those discharged are,

		Males	Females	Total
Males, 110	Cured,	37	71	108
Females, 153	Uncured,			100
———	Unfit from various causes,			28
263	Dead,			27
				263

From the above, it appears, that the proportion of males to females admitted, is nearly as 2 to 3; of females cured to males, nearly as 2 to 1*.

Bethlem Hospital, (commonly called Bedlam,) was appropriated by Henry VIII. to the reception of lunatics, in 1547, at the suppression of monasteries. The present building was completed in 1676. It can contain 170 curable patients on an average Of incurables, it receives 100; fifty of each sex. A new hospital is about building. The improper practice of allowing admission to visitors, has been strictly forbidden and prevented since the year 1770. Physician, Dr. Thomas Munro.

Report of Patients in Bethlem Hospital, Dec. 31, 1809.

Remaining, Dec. 31, 1808,	-	-	-	-	-	147
Admitted in 1809,	-	-	-	-	-	103
						250
Cured and discharged,	-	-	-	-	-	97
Died,	-	-	-	-	-	10
Patients, Dec. 31, 1809,	-	-	-	-	-	143
						250

Of these, men under cure,	-	-	-	-	39	
Incurable,	-	-	-	-	38	
						77	
Women under cure,	-	-	-	-	21	
Incurable,	-	-	-	-	45	
						66	
						143†	

Mr. Haslam states, that from 1748, to 1794, forty-six years, there have been admitted into Bethlem Hospital, 4832 women, and 4042 men. Of the women, 1402 have been discharged cured; and of the men, 1155. The following is a statement of the difference of age in the patients admitted, from 1784 to 1794, ten years.

* Highmore on the Public Charities of London, p. 172.; and Ed. M. & S. J. vol. 4. p. 138.

† Highmore, p. 13. et Seq. & Literary Panorama, vol. 8. p. 870.

Age between	No. admitted.	No. discharged cured.	No. discharged uncured.
10 & 20	113	78	35
20 & 30	488	200	288
30 & 40	527	180	347
40 & 50	362	87	275
50 & 60	143	25	118
60 & 70	31	4	27
	1664	574	1090*

Several other asylums and mad-houses are established in different parts of England. A system of reform on this point, and the erection of hospitals in various central parts of the kingdom, has been proposed by the Committee of the House of Commons, and it is hoped will be adopted. According to their Report, it appears that there were, in July 1807, thirty-seven lunatics confined in different jails; 1878 in houses of correction, poor-houses, &c.; and 483 in private custody; besides about 600 in the public hospitals of London; making nearly 3000 in England alone. The real number, however, is much greater†. In Scotland and Ireland, no public provision has yet been made for them.

FRANCE.

Asylum De Bicêtre. This hospital admits 200 patients. Of these the idiots constitute always one-fourth, if not more. At my last survey, says Mr. Pinel, there were 27 melancholics, 95 maniacs, 18 affected with dementia, and 60 idiots.

* Haslam, p. 245—249.

† Literary Panorama, vol. 2. p. 1259.; and Dr. Willan's Reports on the Diseases of London. He estimates the lunatics in and near London alone, at two thousand.

Maniacs admitted from 1784 to 1794, inclusive, with their respective ages.

	Between 10 & 20	20 & 30	30 & 40	40 & 50	50 & 60	60 & 70	Total.
In 1784	5	33	31	24	11	6	110
1785	4	39	49	25	14	3	134
1786	4	31	40	32	15	5	127
1787	12	39	41	26	17	7	142
1788	9	43	53	21	18	7	151
1789	6	38	39	33	14	2	132
1790	6	28	34	19	9	7	103
1791	9	26	32	16	7	3	93
1792	6	26	33	18	12	3	98
1793	1	13	13	7	4	2	40
1794	3	23	15	15	9	6	71
Total.	65	339	380	236	130	51	1201

The deaths in 1784, were fifty-seven: and in 1788 were ninety-five. In 1794, when the allowance of bread had been raised, they were only twenty-seven*.

Asylum De Charenton. During twenty-two months, 97 patients were admitted; and of these 14 died, and 33 were cured. Out of 71 cases, whose causes could be ascertained, 5 arose from excessive pleasure, 7 from disappointed love, 31 from domestic misfortunes, 1 from terror, 2 from suppressed discharges, 1 from excessive evacuations, and 5 from hereditary predisposition. Physician, Dr. Gastaldi†.

Asylum La Sálpètriere. Dr. Pinel, in less than four years, cured 444, out of 814 maniacs, confined in this hospital. Of 36 struck with accidental madness, 29 recovered‡.

AUSTRIA.

The general hospital at *Vienna*, was founded by Joseph II. and consists of 111 rooms. To it is attached a Lunatic Asylum, of three stories high, each 28 rooms. The shape of the latter is that of a perfectly round tower, but the elevation was probably more to gratify the Emperor's whim, than from any particular advantage resulting from such a structure.

* Pinel on Insanity, p. 32. 112. 173. & 210.
† Pinel, p. 249.
‡ Med. Repository, vol. 12. p. 294.

	Males.	Females.
Remaining at the end of 1804,	170	144
Admitted in 1805, - - - -	117	94
	287	238
Discharged, - - - - -	104	70
Died, - - - - - -	42	32
Remaining at the end of 1805,	141	136
	287	238

The proportion of males to females would probably be greater, were it not for the circumstance of the Ecclesiastics having an asylum for lunatics of their own order*.

PRUSSIA.

The principal hospital for the reception of the sick poor at Berlin, is called, " *La Maison de Charité.*" It is a large building, three stories high, containing about 1200 beds, for three classes of patients, who are separated into three divisions. 1. Medical and surgical cases. 2. Lunatics. 3. Lying-in women, and their children. The clebrated *Hufeland* is superintendant of the Hospital. The following is the number of cases during four years.

	1801	1802	1803	1804
Mental derangement,	179	200	238	200

Under this head is placed all patients affected with mania, melancholia, and fatuitas. The proportion of men to women is as 104 to 56. Out of 334 cases, 105 were cured ; and the cure is said to be owing to the external application of cold water†.

SPAIN.

According to the Rev. Mr. Townsend, the government returns of that country for 1787, gave the following list of lunatics in confinement, in the different provinces.—
Arragon, 244. Valencia, 121. Granada, 41. Leon, 2. Catalonia, 114. Andalusia, 99. Toledo, 42. Avila, 1.
No mention is made of any in the interior provinces‡.

SWITZERLAND.

There are five hospitals in and near Bern, one of which is an asylum for lunatics. Nervous diseases are very common throughout the country, and the proportional number of

* Edin. M. & S. Journal, vol. 2. p. 493.   † Edin. M. & S. J. vol. 2. p. 376
‡ Townsend's Travels in Spain, vol. 2 p. 381

epileptic and lunatic patients is much greater. Upwards of 60 were confined in this asylum, in Aug. 1805, all in separate cells, and almost all of them had dark hair and eyes ; and were melancholic .

NEW-YORK HOSPITAL AND ASYLUM.

Until the year 1808, the insane have been confined in the New-York Hospital. It is stated, on the authority of Dr. Hosack, that during a practice of ten years, as one of the physicians of that Institution, he found the disease to have arisen, in the greatest number of cases, from intemperance ; and that in such, the antiphlogistic treatment was found highly useful. The lunatic asylum was opened on the 15th July, 1808. It contains sixty-four rooms, and can accommodate about 70 patients. Physician, Archibald Bruce, M. D. As there has been but one separate Report of this establishment, (for 1810,) it has, for the sake of convenience, been incorporated with those of the hospital.

	Admitted.		Discharged.				
	Remaining of former years.	Admitted during the year.	Cured.	Relieved.	Discharged from various causes.	Died.	Remaining at the end of the year.
1804	11	46	22	5	12	3	15
1805	15	60	30	4	13	8	20
1806	20	68	29		31	7	21
1807	21	47	18	3	19	4	24
1808	24	66	16	10	16	4	44
1809	44	80	22	4	48	8	42
1810	43	90	44	7	16	10	56
	178	457	181	33	155	44	22

	Males.	Females.
Of 153 in the asylum, in 1810, there were	86	49
Cured, - - - - - - -	35	9
Died, - - - - - -	7†	3
Discharged, - - - - - -	10	13
Remaining, Dec. 31, 1810, - - - -	34	24
	86	49

The above Statement is obtained from authentic documents, and partly through the politeness of Mr. Green, clerk of the New-York hospital.

* Edin. M. & S. Journal, vol. 5. p. 254.
† Of these, two died by suicide, and one a few hours after reception.

epileptic and lunatic patients is much greater. Upwards of 60 were confined in this asylum, in Aug. 1805, all in separate cells, and almost all of them had dark hair and eyes ; and were melancholic .

NEW-YORK HOSPITAL AND ASYLUM.

Until the year 1808, the insane have been confined in the New-York Hospital. It is stated, on the authority of Dr. Hosack, that during a practice of ten years, as one of the physicians of that Institution, he found the disease to have arisen, in the greatest number of cases, from intemperance ; and that in such, the antiphlogistic treatment was found highly useful. The lunatic asylum was opened on the 15th July, 1808. It contains sixty-four rooms, and can accommodate about 70 patients. Physician, Archibald Bruce, M. D. As there has been but one separate Report of this establishment, (for 1810,) it has, for the sake of convenience, been incorporated with those of the hospital.

	Admitted.		Discharged.				
	Remaining of former years.	Admitted during the year.	Cured.	Relieved.	Discharged from various causes.	Died.	Remaining at the end of the year.
1804	11	46	22	5	12	3	15
1805	15	60	30	4	13	8	20
1806	20	68	29		31	7	21
1807	21	47	18	3	19	4	24
1808	24	66	16	10	16	4	44
1809	44	80	22	4	48	8	42
1810	43	90	44	7	16	10	56
	178	457	181	33	155	44	22

	Males.	Females.
Of 153 in the asylum, in 1810, there were	86	49
Cured, - - - - - - -	35	9
Died, - - - - - - -	7†	3
Discharged, - - - - - - -	10	13
Remaining, Dec. 31, 1810, - - - -	34	24
	86	49

The above Statement is obtained from authentic documents, and partly through the politeness of Mr. Green, clerk of the New-York hospital.

* Edin. M. & S. Journal, vol. 5. p. 254.
† Of these, two died by suicide, and one a few hours after reception.

FINIS.

	Males.	Females.
Remaining at the end of 1804,	170	144
Admitted in 1805, - - - -	117	94
	287	238
Discharged, - - - - -	104	70
Died, - - - - - -	42	32
Remaining at the end of 1805,	141	136
	287	238

The proportion of males to females would probably be greater, were it not for the circumstance of the Ecclesiastics having an asylum for lunatics of their own order*.

PRUSSIA.

The principal hospital for the reception of the sick poor at Berlin, is called, " *La Maison de Charité.*" It is a large building, three stories high, containing about 1200 beds, for three classes of patients, who are separated into three divisions. 1. Medical and surgical cases. 2. Lunatics. 3. Lying-in women, and their children. The clebrated *Hufeland* is superintendant of the Hospital. The following is the number of cases during four years.

	1801	1802	1803	1804
Mental derangement,	179	200	238	200

Under this head is placed all patients affected with mania, melancholia, and fatuitas. The proportion of men to women is as 104 to 56. Out of 334 cases, 105 were cured ; and the cure is said to be owing to the external application of cold water†.

SPAIN.

According to the Rev. Mr. Townsend, the government returns of that country for 1787, gave the following list of lunatics in confinement, in the different provinces.—
Arragon, 244. Valencia, 121. Granada, 41. Leon, 2.
Catalonia, 114. Andalusia, 99. Toledo, 42. Avila, 1.
No mention is made of any in the interior provinces‡.

SWITZERLAND.

There are five hospitals in and near Bern, one of which is an asylum for lunatics. Nervous diseases are very common throughout the country, and the proportional number of

* Edin. M. & S. Journal, vol. 2. p. 493. † Edin. M. & S. J. vol. 2. p. 376
‡ Townsend's Travels in Spain, vol. 2. p. 381

MENTAL ILLNESS AND SOCIAL POLICY
THE AMERICAN EXPERIENCE

AN ARNO PRESS COLLECTION

Galt, John M. The Treatment of Insanity. 1846

Goddard, Henry Herbert. Feeble-mindedness: Its Causes and Consequences. 1926

Hammond, William A. A Treatise on Insanity in Its Medical Relations. 1883

Hazard, Thomas R. Report on the Poor and Insane in Rhode-Island. 1851

Hurd, Henry M., editor. The Institutional Care of the Insane in the United States and Canada. 1916/1917. Four volumes.

Kirkbride, Thomas S. On the Construction, Organization, and General Arrangements of Hospitals for the Insane. 1880

Meyer, Adolf. The Commonsense Psychiatry of Dr. Adolf Meyer: Fifty-two Selected Papers. 1948

Mitchell, S. Weir. Wear and Tear, or Hints for the Overworked. 1887

Morton, Thomas G. The History of the Pennsylvania Hospital, 1751-1895. 1895

Ordronaux, John. Jurisprudence in Medicine in Relation to the Law. 1869

The Origins of the State Mental Hospital in America: Six Documentary Studies, 1837-1856. 1973

Packard, Mrs. E. P. W. Modern Persecution, or Insane Asylums Unveiled, As Demonstrated by the Report of the Investigating Committee of the Legislature of Illinois. 1875. Two volumes in one

Prichard, James C. A Treatise on Insanity and Other Disorders Affecting the Mind. 1837

Prince, Morton. The Unconscious: The Fundamentals of Human Personality Normal and Abnormal. 1921

Putnam, James Jackson. Human Motives. 1915

Russell, William Logie. The New York Hospital: A History of the Psychiatric Service, 1771-1936. 1945

Sidis, Boris. The Psychology of Suggestion: A Research into the Subconscious Nature of Man and Society. 1899

Southard, Elmer E. Shell-Shock and Other Neuropsychiatric Problems Presented in Five Hundred and Eighty-Nine Case Histories from the War Literature, 1914-1918. 1919

Southard, E[lmer] E. and Mary C. Jarrett. The Kingdom of Evils. 1922

Southard, E[lmer] E. and H[arry] C. Solomon. Neurosyphilis: Modern Systematic Diagnosis and Treatment Presented in One Hundred and Thirty-seven Case Histories. 1917

Spitzka, E[dward] C. Insanity: Its Classification, Diagnosis and Treatment. 1887

Supreme Court Holding a Criminal Term, No. 14056. The United States vs. Charles J. Guiteau. 1881/1882. Two volumes

Trezevant, Daniel H. Letters to his Excellency Governor Manning on the Lunatic Asylum. 1854

Tuke, D[aniel] Hack. The Insane in the United States and Canada. 1885

Upham, Thomas C. Outlines of Imperfect and Disordered Mental Action. 1868

White, William A[lanson]. Twentieth Century Psychiatry: Its Contribution to Man's Knowledge of Himself. 1936

Willard, Sylvester D. Report on the Condition of the Insane Poor in the County Poor Houses of New York. 1865